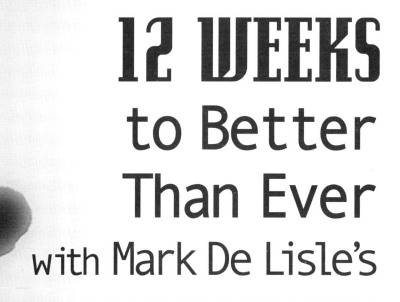

12 WEEKS
to Better
Than Ever
with Mark De Lisle's

NAVY SEAL
BREAKTHROUGH TO
MASTER LEVEL
FITNESS™

Strength
& Honor

BRONZE
BOW PUB.

Disclaimer

The exercises and advice contained within this book may be too strenuous or dangerous for some people, and the reader should consult a physician before engaging in them.

The author and publisher of this book are not responsible in any manner whatsoever for any injury that may occur through reading and following the instructions herein.

"Special thanks to Lor Pace and Lance Wubbels
for making this 12-week program happen."

—Mark De Lisle

CONTENTS

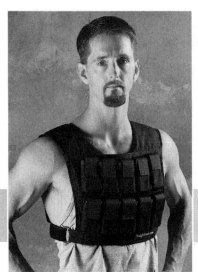

"Change is never easy. . . .
However, for those of us who
truly want to succeed, we must
push ourselves to the next level."

INTRODUCTION

Health, fitness, and quality of life are becoming more and more important to each of us on a daily basis, regardless of where we are currently on the time line of life. We all know that we want to look and feel younger, but in order to do so we must experience a paradigm shift, or in other words, a lifestyle change.

Sadly, change is never easy, which is why most people wander through life with little to no excitement in their daily lives. However, for those of us who truly want to succeed, we must push ourselves to the next level.

This workbook is designed to help you accomplish this very task, and is a companion to the book entitled *Mark De Lisle's Navy SEAL Breakthrough to Master Level Fitness!* Having been a Navy SEAL and a professional fitness trainer, I know this program will take you there.

Like any tool, this workout is only as good as the person using it . . . YOU!

As a result, I have designed this workout to be as simple as possible, cover all of the major components of the book, and yet give you the most complete and comprehensive workout available on the market today.

Unfortunately, there are no magic pills if you are looking for long-term results. However, with dedication and hard work, you can reach your goals and regain the body of your youth. For those who are already "in shape," get ready, because now you are going to push yourself even further than before!

As you use this workbook, you will record your current status, set goals for change, make a plan of action, and then finally complete your transformation to a better, healthier you by finishing the program.

Remember, you can get as much or as little out of this program as you like. Every exercise, every measurement, and every step to your "lifestyle change" is up to you to execute for perfection.

In other words, if you only perform 50% of the program each day, then you can expect 50% of the results. The only person who will suffer is you. Make the decision today to not stop until you reach your goals!

> **Before beginning this body-changing program, make sure you have clearance from your healthcare provider.**

1

FIRST THINGS FIRST

"As you execute this program, do not become discouraged. Permanent change takes time."

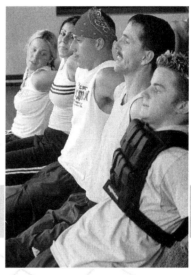

1. READ THE BOOK

In order to maximize the benefit of your "lifestyle change," you must first read the book *Mark De Lisle's Navy SEAL Breakthrough to Master Level Fitness!*

My book will give you insight and instruction on proper form, as well as pictures and demonstrations on the stretches, and exercises necessary to complete this program.

The book also gives the "Why" for doing so many of the different requirements outlined in this workbook. Once you have read Mark's book, and feel that you have a clear understanding, it will be time to start this program.

2. FIND A PARTNER OR GROUP

As you execute this program, do not become discouraged. Permanent change takes time. There will be days when you will not want to work out.

The best solution for combating failure and ensuring your success is to do this program with someone else or a group of people. You will find as you work with others, they will push you toward your goals, and you in turn will push them toward theirs. Through teamwork and the synergistic motivation of others around you, you will see great success with this program!

3. BE PREPARED FOR CHANGE

Remember, this program is a total body workout. It will focus not only on proper exercise, but hydration and nutrition as well. Exercise is not enough. It is only one piece of the entire puzzle. We not only want you to be more fit, we also want you to be healthier.

As you begin to feel better about yourself, it will spill over into the other areas of your life, because success begets success!

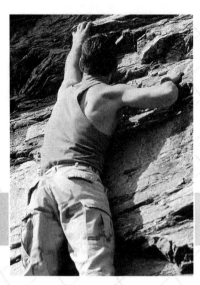

"Keep in mind, people who are lean and mean are that way for a reason...."

2

YOU ARE WHAT YOU EAT

1. EAT RIGHT

Regrettably, most people do not eat healthy. When they become overweight, they diet (starve their bodies) to shed the unwanted pounds. As a result, their bodies store the excess fat from the unhealthy food they eat, or it creates fat and keeps it in storage for the times of famine (dieting). In either scenario, the body is not working optimally.

Keep in mind, people who are lean and mean are that way for a reason. *If looking and feeling younger is one of your goals, then exercise is not enough.* You must make conscious choices regarding your eating habits, by replacing old habits with new ones.

2. SPOIL YOURSELF ONCE A WEEK

"Does eating right mean I have to suffer?" No, not really. In fact, you will find that the more fit you become, the less you will want to eat certain foods. With all the blood, sweat, and tears from your daily workouts, you won't want to throw away all your progress on a doughnut.

"Does that mean that I can't eat what I want?" No, you can . . . Once a week! That's right! Although eat-ing right all the time is the best solution, carrots and celery will never replace a big bowl of ice cream or a chocolate bar!

The point is this. During the week you must stay focused. You must work out on a daily basis and eat properly. *On Saturday or Sunday (not both days), reward yourself with some of life's delicacies.* But, come Monday, it's back to work again.

3. EAT SMALL AND EARLY

In addition to eating properly (foods low in fat), when and how much you eat are also critical.

It is best to eat five small meals throughout the day, and whenever possible NO FOOD 4 hours prior to going to bed at night.

Imagine your stomach as a furnace that runs more efficiently if it is constantly burning. If you rarely add fuel to burn, or you put in too much fuel at a time, the furnace will not function properly. On the other hand, if the furnace is always burning and is never overworked, your stomach will digest food faster and more efficiently. *Our bodies have a hard time using poorly digested food, and usually convert it to fat.*

4. DRINK PLENTY OF WATER

Equally as important to eating right is hydration. Most people do not drink enough water. On average, a person should drink 8 ten-ounce glasses of water a day. Water is critical for circulating the necessary nutrients into one's cells, as well as eliminating toxins and waste from the body. Water is also needed to keep our bodies from overheating. *Remember, when you feel thirsty, you are already dehydrated! Don't wait until you get to this point.*

5. SUPPLEMENT YOUR DIET

Eating right isn't enough anymore. Sadly, even some of our best foods are not enriched with the same amount of vitamins and minerals of even a generation ago. As a result, *it is necessary to supplement one's diet with those nutrients necessary for proper health.* I recommend the following IONYX supplements for meeting one's daily minimums, and IONYX has created a fit pak specifically designed to provide daily support for my workout. Check it out on page 54.

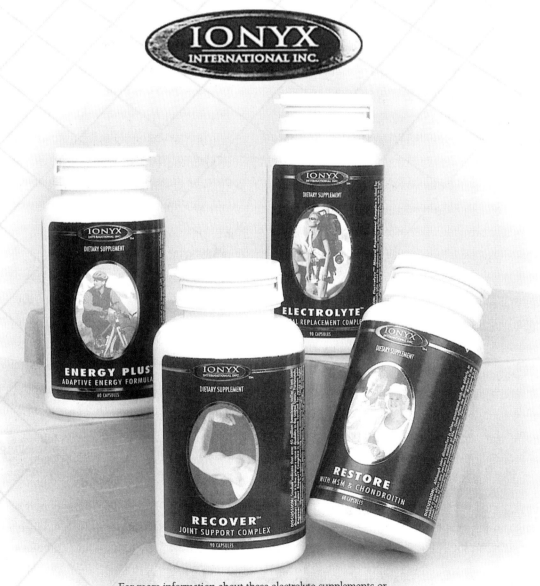

For more information about these electrolyte supplements or
to find out how to purchase IONYX products, please refer to my
Web site at www.masterlevelfitness.com.

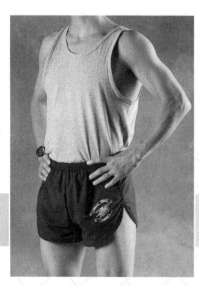

"After all, isn't it going to be fantastic when you feel and look younger again!"

3

MY BEFORE BODY...

1. MEASURE YOUR BODY

As is the case in most of life's many experiences, it is just as important to know where you have been, as it is to know where you are going. So for the last time, we need to take a good hard look at your current body.

Although it may be a little uncomfortable, we suggest that you use your partner for this chapter. "WHY?" It's simple. *You need to record your measurements, and it is easier for someone else to measure your body for you.*

Remember, your loved ones want you to be healthy. They want you to succeed, and if you let them, they can even help you. So, don't let discomfort keep you from reaching your goals! Let your loved ones give you the encouragement and support necessary for you to obtain that body that you have temporarily misplaced!

A little bit of embarrassment is a good thing. If anything, it will give you more encouragement to make the change.

2. TAKE PICTURES OF YOUR BODY

Have your partner take your "before body" pictures, to visually record your transformation! When taking your pictures, you will need full-length, frontal, side, and backside views of your body. For the best results, make sure you use a well-lit room, and, if possible, wear a swimsuit or other clothing that will expose your "before body."

Keep in mind that at the end of the program, you will also take pictures of your "new body!" You may also want to track your progress. *Post your pictures somewhere that will remind you of your motivation!*

3. WEIGHT DOESN'T MATTER

During your beginning stages, you may want to track your weight, because you will be shedding unwanted fat. However, there will come a point where you will start putting on weight again . . . this is great, because muscle weighs more than fat! As a result, *your end goal shouldn't be how much you weigh, but rather how you feel and look.*

One of the main reasons for taking your measurements is because everyone loses weight differently, and in different parts of their bodies. By tracking your measurements, you will see progress that you might not have noticed as quickly (i.e., In the beginning you may only lose a few pounds, which may not seem like much, but your measurements show that those few pounds equate to 4 inches off of your waist . . . not bad.). Remember to celebrate your successes!

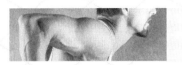

MY MEASUREMENTS

	Date	Weight	Neck	Shoulders	Biceps (flexed)	Chest (relaxed)	Chest (flexed)	Waist	Hips (females)	Thighs	Calves
Start	/ /										
End of Week 1	/ /										
End of Week 2	/ /										
End of Week 3	/ /										
End of Week 4	/ /										
End of Week 5	/ /										
End of Week 6	/ /										
End of Week 7	/ /										
End of Week 8	/ /										
End of Week 9	/ /										
End of Week 10	/ /										
End of Week 11	/ /										
End of Week 12	/ /										
− Start											
= + or −											

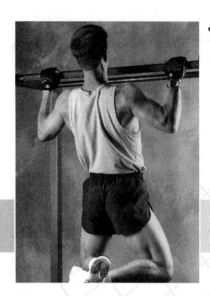

"Do not sacrifice form for repetitions.
You will only be cheating yourself!"

4

READY...

1. SET YOUR FITNESS LEVEL

In order to optimize this program, you must prepare by benchmarking your current fitness level. Remember this is only a starting point. Once you begin your training, you may need to adjust (increase or decrease) your repetitions or move to a higher level until you are maximizing your workout (the best time for setting your benchmark is on the Saturday before you begin working out).

When creating your benchmark, perform every exercise outlined on the following page. Each exercise must be done to exhaustion (usually within a 2-minute period).

When performing each exercise, make sure you maintain the proper form at all times. This must be done for a variety of reasons. First, each exercise is specifically chosen to target a specific part of the body. Second, improper form can cause injury.

As you perform each exercise, you will create "snap shots" of your current physical fitness for a given part of the body.

Do not become discouraged if you do not have the same fitness level as someone else. Everyone's starting point is different.

2. BE HONEST

As you take your evaluation test, you may find that in four of the five areas you are a beginner, but in the fifth area you are advanced. This is okay. Once you start your weekly routines, you need to exercise each body part at the level it is challenged.

Remember, your fitness evaluation is a guide for your weekly workouts; therefore, you need an honest view of your current fitness levels. As a result, *do not sacrifice form for repetitions. You will only be cheating yourself.*

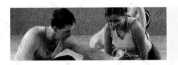

FITNESS EVALUATION

Use this fitness evaluation as a general overall look at your fitness level. Record the maximum number of repetitions for each of the following exercises, then check the corresponding box for the level of the exercise you performed. When you begin your workout, use the correct fitness level for each exercise as a starting point. Adjust reps and pyramids as necessary or move to a higher level whenever possible.

EXERCISES (Regular)	Total Max Reps	Beginning Level	Intermediate Level	Advanced Level
Push-Ups		32	72	130
Crunches		20	50	100
Lunges		10	25	50
Bar Dips		10	20	30
Flutter Kicks		20	40	60
Calf Raises		75	90	120

Choose the corresponding level and stage from the following pyramid tables as a guide when performing upper body workouts.

EXERCISES		Beginning Level		Intermediate Level		Advanced Level	
		Stage 1	Stage 2	Stage 3	Stage 4	Stage 5	Stage 6
PUSH-UPS	Regular	2-4-2	2-4-6-4-2	2-4-6-8-10-8-6-4-2	4-6-8-10-12-10-8-6-4	6-8-10-12-14-12-10-8-6	8-10-12-14-16-14-12-10-8
	Diamond	2-4-2	2-4-6-4-2	2-4-6-8-6-4-2	2-4-6-8-10-8-6-4-2	4-6-8-10-12-10-8-6-4	8-10-12-14-12-10-8
	Dive Bombers	2-4-2	2-4-6-4-2	2-4-6-8-6-4-2	2-4-6-8-10-8-6-4-2	4-6-8-10-12-10-8-6-4	8-10-12-14-12-10-8
PULL-UPS	Regular	2-4-2	2-4-6-4-2	2-4-6-8-6-4-2	2-4-6-8-10-8-6-4-2	4-6-8-10-12-10-8-6-4	8-10-12-14-12-10-8
	Close Grip	1-2-1	1-2-4-2-1	2-4-6-4-2	2-4-6-8-6-4-2	2-4-6-8-10-8-6-4-2	4-6-8-10-12-10-8-6-4
	Reverse Grip	1-2-1	1-2-4-2-1	2-4-6-4-2	2-4-6-8-6-4-2	2-4-6-8-10-8-6-4-2	4-6-8-10-12-10-8-6-4
	Commandos	1-1-1	1-2-1	1-2-4-2-1	2-4-6-4-2	4-6-8-6-4	4-6-8-10-8-6-4
	Behind the Neck	1-2-1	1-2-1	1-2-4-2-1	2-4-6-4-2	4-6-8-6-4	4-6-8-10-8-6-4

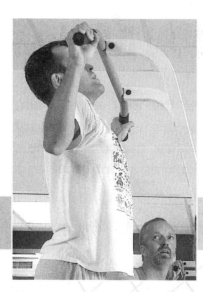

"Goals keep you focused on the end results and are necessary for true commitment."

5

AIM...

1. VISUALIZE YOUR FUTURE

What kind of body do you want to have in 90 days? Cut out pictures and post them in conspicuous places where you will see them. *Imagine yourself with your new body.* (You may even want to place your face on the pictures of your future body.)

2. SET REALISTIC GOALS

In order to obtain your sculpted body, you must set goals. Goals keep you focused on the end results and are necessary for true commitment. *If you are not committed, you will fail. Your goals must also be realistic or you will also fail.*

First, set your 90 day goals. Second, break these goals into monthly segments, by dividing these goals by 3. Then divide your monthly goals by 4 to set your weekly goals.

As you break down your goals into smaller pieces, they are much easier to attain. Each time you reach your smaller goals, it will give you the confidence and assurance you need to reach your final goals.

3. REWARD YOURSELF

Although in many cases your "new body" is reward enough, we want you to go the extra mile, by giving yourself a special reward for meeting your goals.

Your reward might be a vacation to an exotic place where you can wear a new swimsuit. Maybe there is a smaller dress size or outfit that you have your eye on buying or a new set of golf clubs, a boat, or tools. Regardless, *give yourself a prize for accomplishing your goals. You have worked hard and you deserve it!*

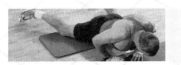 # "NEW BODY" GOALS

90 DAY GOALS

1. _____

2. _____

3. _____

4. _____

MONTHLY GOALS (Divide 90 day goals by 3)

1. _____

2. _____

3. _____

4. _____

WEEKLY GOALS (Divide monthly goals by 4)

1. _____

2. _____

3. _____

4. _____

REWARDS

SHORT-TERM (After 30 Days) _____

MID-TERM (After 45 Days) _____

LONG-TERM (After 90 Days) _____

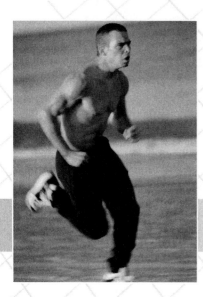

"There is no reason
for further procrastination.
The time is NOW!"

6

FIRE!

1. TIME TO TAKE OFF

Normally, when a person yells "FIRE!" in a building, people jump out of their seats and take off running for their lives. . . .

Well, consider this a FIRE, and start running as if your life depends on it, by putting everything you have learned into action!

2. THERE'S NO LOOKING BACK

By now, you have read and understand the book *Mark De Lisle's Navy SEAL Breakthrough to Master Level Fitness!*

There is no reason for further procrastination. The time is NOW! Don't put off any longer what you know you have to do. Decide today that you are will-ing to meet the goals you have set, regardless of what may come up in the next 90 days. *Commit yourself to*

changing your body. As the Navy SEAL would say, "Dig deep, and use your fire in the gut" to make those changes that will alter your lifestyle forever.

Change your eating habits, drink more water, eat less before going to bed. Constantly visualize your new body, and how your life is already changing for the better.

Review your goals. Look at the pictures of your future body that you have posted around your house, and remember the reward that you will be giving yourself for all your hard work.

3. YOU ARE IN CONTROL

You can change your life. You have the tools, desire, and ability to succeed. *In 90 days you will have a new body, because you are in control of your future.* We look forward to seeing and hearing of your successes.

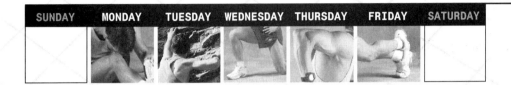

| SUNDAY | MONDAY | TUESDAY | WEDNESDAY | THURSDAY | FRIDAY | SATURDAY |

THE PROGRAM

BEGINNING LEVEL

INTERMEDIATE LEVEL

ADVANCED LEVEL

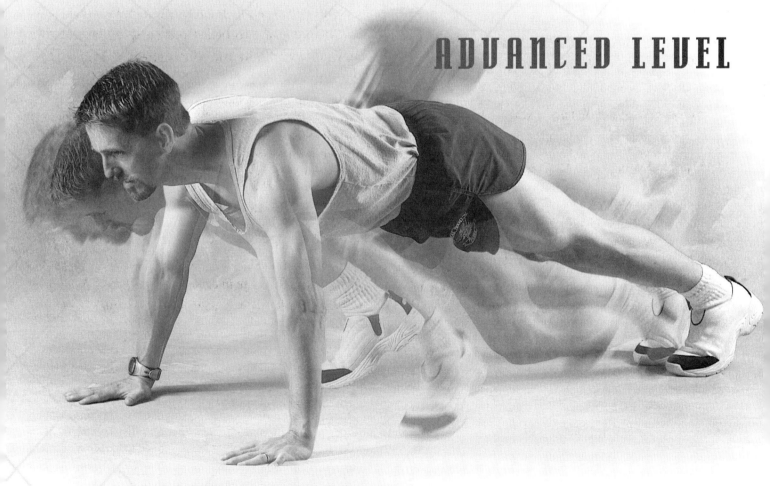

WEEK 1   BEGINNING LEVEL

✓ MONDAY / /	✓ TUESDAY / /	✓ WEDNESDAY / /	✓ THURSDAY / /	✓ FRIDAY / /
Take "Before" Supplements	Take "Before" Supplements	Take "Before" Supplements	Take "Before" Supplements	Take "Before" Supplements
Drink 16 oz. of water	Drink 16 oz. of water	Drink 16 oz. of water	Drink 16 oz. of water	Drink 16 oz. of water
WARM-UPS	**WARM-UPS**	**WARM-UPS**	**WARM-UPS**	**WARM-UPS**
Jumping Jacks 25	Jumping Jacks 30	Jumping Jacks 25	Jumping Jacks 30	Jumping Jacks 25
Running in Place 30 sec.	Running in Place 30 sec.	Running in Place 30 sec.	Running in Place 30 sec.	Running in Place 30 sec.
Half Jumping Jacks 25	Half Jumping Jacks 30	Half Jumping Jacks 25	Half Jumping Jacks 30	Half Jumping Jacks 25
60–90 sec. Rest	60–90 sec. Rest	60–90 sec. Rest	60–90 sec. Rest	60–90 sec. Rest
STRETCHES	**STRETCHES**	**LEGS**	**STRETCHES**	**STRETCHES**
Bend Overs	Chest	Walking Lunges 20 yds. (2x)	Chest	Bend Overs
Cross Overs	Lat	High Knees 20 yds. (2x)	Lat	Cross Overs
Inner Thigh	Shoulders	Frog Hops 20 yds. (2x)	Shoulders	Inner Thigh
Forward Lunge	Tricep	Star Hops 10	Tricep	Forward Lunge
Side & Oblique	Partner	Mountain Climbers 10	Partner	Side & Oblique
Hurdler	Arm Rotation	**SPRINTS**	Arm Rotation	Hurdler
Butterfly	60–90 sec. Rest	Intervals (Optional)	60–90 sec. Rest	Butterfly
ITB	**UPPER BODY**	2 Laps = 800 yds.	**UPPER BODY**	ITB
Thigh	Neck Rotations 10		Neck Rotations 10	Thigh
Calf	Back Contractions 10		Back Contractions 10	Calf
60–90 sec. Rest	Swimmer Exercise 10		Swimmer Exercise 10	60–90 sec. Rest
LEGS	Back Lifts 10		Back Lifts 10	**LEGS**
Lunges 10	60–90 sec. Rest		60–90 sec. Rest	Lunges 10
Squats 20	**PULL-UPS**		**PULL-UPS**	Squats 20
Fire Hydrants 10 (Each Side)	Regular 2-4-2		Regular 2-4-2	Fire Hydrants 10 (Each Side)
Mountain Climber 10	Close Grip 1-2-1		Close Grip 1-2-1	Mountain Climber 10
The Wall 1 min.	Reverse 1-2-1		Reverse 1-2-1	The Wall 1 min.
60–90 sec. Rest	Commandos 1-1-1		Commandos 1-1-1	60–90 sec. Rest
CALVES	Behind the Neck 1-2-1		Behind the Neck 1-2-1	**CALVES**
Straight (Regular) 50	60–90 sec. Rest		60–90 sec. Rest	Straight (Regular) 50
Toe to Toe 50	**BAR DIPS**		**BAR DIPS**	Toe to Toe 50
Heel to Heel 50	Regular 5 (4 sets)		Regular	Heel to Heel 50
60–90 sec. Rest	60–90 sec. Rest		60–90 sec. Rest	60–90 sec. Rest
ABDOMINALS	**PUSH-UPS**		**PUSH-UPS**	**ABDOMINALS**
Hand to Toes 10	Regular 2-4-6-8-6-4-2	**ABDOMINALS**	Regular 2-4-6-8-6-4-2	Hand to Toes 10
X Sit-Ups 10	Diamond 2-4-6-4-2	Clockwork 15-10-5	Diamond 2-4-6-4-2	X Sit-Ups 10
Crunches 10	Dive Bombers 2-4-6-4-2	Hanging Knee Up 10	Dive Bombers 2-4-6-4-2	Crunches 10
Side Sit-Ups 10	8 Count Body Builders 5	Hanging Side Sit-Up 5	8 Count Body Builders 5	Side Sit-Ups 10
Obliques 10	Take "After" Supplements	Hand to Toe (Short) 10	Take "After" Supplements	Obliques 10
Flutter Kicks 10	Drink 16 oz. of water	Crunches (Short) 10	Drink 16 oz. of water	Flutter Kicks 10
Reverse Crunches 10		Side Sit-Up (Short) 10		Reverse Crunches 10
Knee Bends 10		Obliques (Short) 10		Knee Bends 10
Chest Roll		Take "After" Supplements		Chest Roll 10
Take "After" Supplements		Drink 16 oz. of water		Take "After" Supplements
Drink 16 oz. of water				Drink 1 quart of water

MONDAY

MEALS   **WATER**
1 2 3 4 | 1 2 3 4
5 | 5 6 7 8

SUPPLEMENTS

Before	After
3 Electrolyte™	**3** Recover™
1 Energy Plus™	**2** Restore™

TUESDAY

MEALS   **WATER**
1 2 3 4 | 1 2 3 4
5 | 5 6 7 8

SUPPLEMENTS

Before	After
3 Electrolyte™	**3** Recover™
1 Energy Plus™	**2** Restore™

WEDNESDAY

MEALS   **WATER**
1 2 3 4 | 1 2 3 4
5 | 5 6 7 8

SUPPLEMENTS

Before	After
3 Electrolyte™	**3** Recover™
1 Energy Plus™	**2** Restore™

THURSDAY

MEALS   **WATER**
1 2 3 4 | 1 2 3 4
5 | 5 6 7 8

SUPPLEMENTS

Before	After
3 Electrolyte™	**3** Recover™
1 Energy Plus™	**2** Restore™

FRIDAY

MEALS   **WATER**
1 2 3 4 | 1 2 3 4
5 | 5 6 7 8

SUPPLEMENTS

Before	After
3 Electrolyte™	**3** Recover™
1 Energy Plus™	**2** Restore™

WEEK 2   BEGINNING LEVEL

✓ MONDAY / /	✓ TUESDAY / /	✓ WEDNESDAY / /	✓ THURSDAY / /	✓ FRIDAY / /
Take "Before" Supplements	Take "Before" Supplements	Take "Before" Supplements	Take "Before" Supplements	Take "Before" Supplements
Drink 16 oz. of water	Drink 16 oz. of water	Drink 16 oz. of water	Drink 16 oz. of water	Drink 16 oz. of water
WARM-UPS	**WARM-UPS**	**WARM-UPS**	**WARM-UPS**	**WARM-UPS**
Jumping Jacks 25	Jumping Jacks 30	Jumping Jacks 25	Jumping Jacks 30	Jumping Jacks 25
Running in Place 30 sec.	Running in Place 30 sec.	Running in Place 30 sec.	Running in Place 30 sec.	Running in Place 30 sec.
Half Jumping Jacks 25	Half Jumping Jacks 30	Half Jumping Jacks 25	Half Jumping Jacks 30	Half Jumping Jacks 25
60–90 sec. Rest	60–90 sec. Rest	60–90 sec. Rest	60–90 sec. Rest	60–90 sec. Rest
STRETCHES	**STRETCHES**	**LEGS**	**STRETCHES**	**STRETCHES**
Bend Overs	Chest	Walking Lunges 20 yds. (2x)	Chest	Bend Overs
Cross Overs	Lat	High Knees 20 yds. (2x)	Lat	Cross Overs
Inner Thigh	Shoulders	Frog Hops 20 yds. (2x)	Shoulders	Inner Thigh
Forward Lunge	Tricep	Star Hops 10	Tricep	Forward Lunge
Side & Oblique	Partner	Mountain Climbers 10	Partner	Side & Oblique
Hurdler	Arm Rotation	**SPRINTS**	Arm Rotation	Hurdler
Butterfly	60–90 sec. Rest	Basic Sprints (Optional)	60–90 sec. Rest	Butterfly
ITB	**UPPER BODY**	800 yd. Warm-Up	**UPPER BODY**	ITB
Thigh	Neck Rotations 20	3 Sets of Cones	Neck Rotations 20	Thigh
Calf	Back Contractions 20	First Set — 50%	Back Contractions 20	Calf
60–90 sec. Rest	Swimmer Exercise 10	Second Set — 75%	Swimmer Exercise 10	60–90 sec. Rest
LEGS	Back Lifts 10	Third Set — 100%	Back Lifts 10	**LEGS**
Lunges 13	60–90 sec. Rest	5 Sets	60–90 sec. Rest	Lunges 13
Squats 23	**PULL-UPS**		**PULL-UPS**	Squats 23
Fire Hydrants 11 (Each Side)	Regular 2-4-2		Regular 2-4-2	Fire Hydrants 11 (Each Side)
Mountain Climber 10	Close Grip 1-2-1		Close Grip 1-2-1	Mountain Climber 10
The Wall 1 min.	Reverse 1-2-1		Reverse 1-2-1	The Wall 1 min.
60–90 sec. Rest	Commandos 1-1-1		Commandos 1-1-1	60–90 sec. Rest
CALVES	Behind the Neck 1-2-1		Behind the Neck 1-2-1	**CALVES**
Straight (Regular) 50	60–90 sec. Rest		60–90 sec. Rest	Straight (Regular) 50
Toe to Toe 50	**BAR DIPS**		**BAR DIPS**	Toe to Toe 50
Heel to Heel 50	Regular 5 (4 sets)		Regular 5 (4 sets)	Heel to Heel 50
60–90 sec. Rest	60–90 sec. Rest		60–90 sec. Rest	60–90 sec. Rest
ABDOMINALS	**PUSH-UPS**		**PUSH-UPS**	**ABDOMINALS**
Hand to Toes 10	Regular 2-4-6-8-6-4-2	**ABDOMINALS**	Regular 2-4-6-8-6-4-2	Hand to Toes 10
X Sit-Ups 10	Diamond 2-4-6-4-2	Clockwork 15-10-5	Diamond 2-4-6-4-2	X Sit-Ups 10
Crunches 10	Dive Bombers 2-4-6-4-2	Hanging Knee Up 10	Dive Bombers 2-4-6-4-2	Crunches 10
Side Sit-Ups 10	8 Count Body Builders 5	Hanging Side Sit-Up 5	8 Count Body Builders 5	Side Sit-Ups 10
Obliques 10	Take "After" Supplements	Hand to Toes (Short) 10	Take "After" Supplements	Obliques 10
Flutter Kicks 10	Drink 16 oz. of water	Crunches (Short) 10	Drink 16 oz. of water	Flutter Kicks 10
Reverse Crunches 10		Side Sit-Up (Short) 10		Reverse Crunches 10
Knee Bends 10		Obliques (Short) 10		Knee Bends 10
Chest Roll 10		Take "After" Supplements		Chest Roll 10
Take "After" Supplements		Drink 16 oz. of water		Take "After" Supplements
Drink 16 oz. of water				Drink 1 quart of water

	MONDAY		TUESDAY		WEDNESDAY		THURSDAY		FRIDAY
MEALS	1 2 3 4 5	**WATER** 1 2 3 4 5 6 7 8	**MEALS** 1 2 3 4 5	**WATER** 1 2 3 4 5 6 7 8	**MEALS** 1 2 3 4 5	**WATER** 1 2 3 4 5 6 7 8	**MEALS** 1 2 3 4 5	**WATER** 1 2 3 4 5 6 7 8	**MEALS** 1 2 3 4 5	**WATER** 1 2 3 4 5 6 7 8

SUPPLEMENTS

	Before	After
Monday	3 Electrolyte™ / 1 Energy Plus™	3 Recover™ / 2 Restore™
Tuesday	3 Electrolyte™ / 1 Energy Plus™	3 Recover™ / 2 Restore™
Wednesday	3 Electrolyte™ / 1 Energy Plus™	3 Recover™ / 2 Restore™
Thursday	3 Electrolyte™ / 1 Energy Plus™	3 Recover™ / 2 Restore™
Friday	3 Electrolyte™ / 1 Energy Plus™	3 Recover™ / 2 Restore™

WEEK 3 — BEGINNING LEVEL

MONDAY / /

- Take "Before" Supplements
- Drink 16 oz. of water

WARM-UPS
- Jumping Jacks 25
- Running in Place 30 sec.
- Half Jumping Jacks 25
- 60–90 sec. Rest

STRETCHES
- Bend Overs
- Cross Overs
- Inner Thigh
- Forward Lunge
- Side & Oblique
- Hurdler
- Butterfly
- ITB
- Thigh
- Calf
- 60–90 sec. Rest

LEGS
- Lunges 16
- Squats 26
- Fire Hydrants 13 (Each Side)
- Mountain Climber 11
- The Wall 1:15 min.
- 60–90 sec. Rest

CALVES
- Straight (Regular) 55
- Toe to Toe 55
- Heel to Heel 55
- 60–90 sec. Rest

ABDOMINALS
- Hand to Toes 11
- X Sit-Ups 11
- Crunches 11
- Side Sit-Ups 11
- Obliques 11
- Flutter Kicks 11
- Reverse Crunches 11
- Knee Bends 11
- Chest Roll 11
- Take "After" Supplements
- Drink 16 oz. of water

TUESDAY / /

- Take "Before" Supplements
- Drink 16 oz. of water

WARM-UPS
- Jumping Jacks 30
- Running in Place 30 sec.
- Half Jumping Jacks 30
- 60–90 sec. Rest

STRETCHES
- Chest
- Lat
- Shoulders
- Tricep
- Partner
- Arm Rotation
- 60–90 sec. Rest

UPPER BODY
- Neck Rotations 22
- Back Contractions 22
- Swimmer Exercise 12
- Back Lifts 11
- 60–90 sec. Rest

PULL-UPS
- Regular 2-4-2
- Close Grip 1-2-1
- Reverse 1-2-1
- Commandos 1-1-1
- Behind the Neck 1-2-3-2-1
- 60–90 sec. Rest

BAR DIPS
- Regular 6
- 60–90 sec. Rest

PUSH-UPS
- Regular 2-4-6-8-6-4-2
- Diamond 2-4-6-4-2
- Dive Bombers 2-4-6-4-2
- 8 Count Body Builders 6
- Take "After" Supplements
- Drink 16 oz. of water

WEDNESDAY / /

- Take "Before" Supplements
- Drink 16 oz. of water

WARM-UPS
- Jumping Jacks 25
- Running in Place 30 sec.
- Half Jumping Jacks 25
- 60–90 sec. Rest

LEGS
- Walking Lunges 25 yds. (2x)
- High Knees 25 yds. (2x)
- Frog Hops 25 yds. (2x)
- Star Hops 10
- Mountain Climbers 10

SPRINTS
- Intervals (Optional)
- 3 Laps = 1200 yds.

ABDOMINALS
- Clockwork 15-10-5
- Hanging Knee Up 11
- Hanging Side Sit-Up 6
- Hand to Toes (Short) 11
- Crunches (Short) 11
- Side Sit-Up (Short) 11
- Obliques (Short) 11
- Take "After" Supplements
- Drink 16 oz. of water

THURSDAY / /

- Take "Before" Supplements
- Drink 16 oz. of water

WARM-UPS
- Jumping Jacks 30
- Running in Place 30 sec.
- Half Jumping Jacks 30
- 60–90 sec. Rest

STRETCHES
- Chest
- Lat
- Shoulders
- Tricep
- Partner
- Arm Rotation
- 60–90 sec. Rest

UPPER BODY
- Neck Rotations 22
- Back Contractions 22
- Swimmer Exercise 12
- Back Lifts 11
- 60–90 sec. Rest

PULL-UPS
- Regular 2-4-2
- Close Grip 1-2-1
- Reverse 1-2-1
- Commandos 1-1-1
- Behind the Neck 1-2-3-2-1
- 60–90 sec. Rest

BAR DIPS
- Regular 6
- 60–90 sec. Rest

PUSH-UPS
- Regular 2-4-6-8-6-4-2
- Diamond 2-4-6-4-2
- Dive Bombers 2-4-6-4-2
- 8 Count Body Builders 6
- Take "After" Supplements
- Drink 16 oz. of water

FRIDAY / /

- Take "Before" Supplements
- Drink 16 oz. of water

WARM-UPS
- Jumping Jacks 25
- Running in Place 30 sec.
- Half Jumping Jacks 25
- 60–90 sec. Rest

STRETCHES
- Bend Overs
- Cross Overs
- Inner Thigh
- Forward Lunge
- Side & Oblique
- Hurdler
- Butterfly
- ITB
- Thigh
- Calf
- 60–90 sec. Rest

LEGS
- Lunges 16
- Squats 26
- Fire Hydrants 13 (Each Side)
- Mountain Climber 11
- The Wall 1:15 min.
- 60–90 sec. Rest

CALVES
- Straight (Regular) 55
- Toe to Toe 55
- Heel to Heel 55
- 60–90 sec. Rest

ABDOMINALS
- Hand to Toes 11
- X Sit-Ups 11
- Crunches 11
- Side Sit-Ups 11
- Obliques 11
- Flutter Kicks 11
- Reverse Crunches 11
- Knee Bends 11
- Chest Roll 11
- Take "After" Supplements
- Drink 1 quart of water

Daily Tracking (each day Monday–Friday)

MEALS: 1 2 3 4 5

WATER: 1 2 3 4 5 6 7 8

SUPPLEMENTS

Before	After
3 Electrolyte™	3 Recover™
1 Energy Plus™	2 Restore™

WEEK 4 — BEGINNING LEVEL

✓ MONDAY / /	✓ TUESDAY / /	✓ WEDNESDAY / /	✓ THURSDAY / /	✓ FRIDAY / /
Take "Before" Supplements	Take "Before" Supplements	Take "Before" Supplements	Take "Before" Supplements	Take "Before" Supplements
Drink 16 oz. of water	Drink 16 oz. of water	Drink 16 oz. of water	Drink 16 oz. of water	Drink 16 oz. of water
WARM-UPS	**WARM-UPS**	**WARM-UPS**	**WARM-UPS**	**WARM-UPS**
Jumping Jacks 25	Jumping Jacks 30	Jumping Jacks 25	Jumping Jacks 30	Jumping Jacks 25
Running in Place 30 sec.	Running in Place 30 sec.	Running in Place 30 sec.	Running in Place 30 sec.	Running in Place 30 sec.
Half Jumping Jacks 25	Half Jumping Jacks 30	Half Jumping Jacks 25	Half Jumping Jacks 30	Half Jumping Jacks 25
60–90 sec. Rest	60–90 sec. Rest	60–90 sec. Rest	60–90 sec. Rest	60–90 sec. Rest
STRETCHES	**STRETCHES**	**LEGS**	**STRETCHES**	**STRETCHES**
Bend Overs	Chest	Walking Lunges 25 yds. (2x)	Chest	Bend Overs
Cross Overs	Lat	High Knees 25 yds. (2x)	Lat	Cross Overs
Inner Thigh	Shoulders	Frog Hops 25 yds. (2x)	Shoulders	Inner Thigh
Forward Lunge	Tricep	Star Hops 12	Tricep	Forward Lunge
Side & Oblique	Partner	Mountain Climbers 12	Partner	Side & Oblique
Hurdler	Arm Rotation	**SPRINTS**	Arm Rotation	Hurdler
Butterfly	60–90 sec. Rest	Basic Sprints (Optional)	60–90 sec. Rest	Butterfly
ITB	**UPPER BODY**	800 yd. Warm-Up	***BURNOUTS— UPPER BODY***	ITB
Thigh	Neck Rotations 24	3 Sets of Cones		Thigh
Calf	Back Contractions 24	First Set — 50%	**SET 1**	Calf
60–90 sec. Rest	Swimmer Exercise 12	Second Set — 75%	Regular Pull-Ups	60–90 sec. Rest
LEGS	Back Lifts 11	Third Set — 100%	Bar Dips	***BURNOUTS— LEGS***
Lunges 19	60–90 sec. Rest	6 Sets	Regular Push-Ups	
Squats 29	**PULL-UPS**		**SET 2**	**SET 1**
Fire Hydrants 15 (Each Side)	Regular 2-4-6-4-2		Close Grip Pull-Ups	The Wall
Mountain Climber 12	Close Grip 2-4-2		Bar Dips	Frog Hops
The Wall 1:15 min.	Reverse 2-4-2		Diamond Push-Ups	Hand to Toe
60–90 sec. Rest	Commandos 1-2-1		**SET 3**	**SET 2**
CALVES	Behind the Neck 1-2-3-2-1		Reverse Grip Pull-Ups	Lunges
Straight (Regular) 55	60–90 sec. Rest		Bar Dips	Star Hops
Toe to Toe 55	**BAR DIPS**		Dive Bombers	Side Sit-Ups
Heel to Heel 55	Regular 6		**SET 4**	**SET 3**
60–90 sec. Rest 55	60–90 sec. Rest		Behind the Neck Pull-Ups	Mountain Climbers
ABDOMINALS	**PUSH-UPS**		Bar Dips	Knee Bends
Hand to Toes 11	Regular 2-4-6-8-6-4-2	**ABDOMINALS**	Regular Push-Ups	**SET 4**
X Sit-Ups 11	Diamond 2-4-6-4-2	Clockwork 15-10-5	**SET 5**	Fire Hydrants (Each Side)
Crunches 11	Dive Bombers 2-4-6-4-2	Hanging Knee Up 11	Commandos	High Knees
Side Sit-Ups 11	8 Count Body Builders 6	Hanging Side Sit-Up 6	Bar Dips	Crunches
Obliques 11	Take "After" Supplements	Hand to Toes (Short) 11	Diamond Push-Ups	**SET 5**
Flutter Kicks 11	Drink 16 oz. of water	Crunches (Short) 11	Take "After" Supplements	Calf Raises
Reverse Crunches 11		Side Sit-Up (Short) 11	Drink 16 oz. of water	Sprints
Knee Bends 11		Obliques (Short) 11		Knee Roll Ups
Chest Roll 11		Atomic 5		Take "After" Supplements
Take "After" Supplements		Take "After" Supplements		Drink 1 quart of water
Drink 16 oz. of water		Drink 16 oz. of water		

MEALS	WATER	MEALS	WATER	MEALS	WATER	MEALS	WATER	MEALS	WATER
1 2 3 4 / 5	1 2 3 4 / 5 6 7 8	1 2 3 4 / 5	1 2 3 4 / 5 6 7 8	1 2 3 4 / 5	1 2 3 4 / 5 6 7 8	1 2 3 4 / 5	1 2 3 4 / 5 6 7 8	1 2 3 4 / 5	1 2 3 4 / 5 6 7 8

SUPPLEMENTS

Before	After	Before	After	Before	After	Before	After	Before	After
3 Electrolyte™ / **1** Energy Plus™	**3** Recover™ / **2** Restore™	**3** Electrolyte™ / **1** Energy Plus™	**3** Recover™ / **2** Restore™	**3** Electrolyte™ / **1** Energy Plus™	**3** Recover™ / **2** Restore™	**3** Electrolyte™ / **1** Energy Plus™	**3** Recover™ / **2** Restore™	**3** Electrolyte™ / **1** Energy Plus™	**3** Recover™ / **2** Restore™

WEEK 5 — BEGINNING LEVEL

✓ MONDAY / /	✓ TUESDAY / /	✓ WEDNESDAY / /	✓ THURSDAY / /	✓ FRIDAY / /
Take "Before" Supplements	Take "Before" Supplements	Take "Before" Supplements	Take "Before" Supplements	Take "Before" Supplements
Drink 16 oz. of water	Drink 16 oz. of water	Drink 16 oz. of water	Drink 16 oz. of water	Drink 16 oz. of water
WARM-UPS	**WARM-UPS**	**WARM-UPS**	**WARM-UPS**	**WARM-UPS**
Jumping Jacks 25	Jumping Jacks 30	Jumping Jacks 25	Jumping Jacks 30	Jumping Jacks 25
Running in Place 30 sec.	Running in Place 30 sec.	Running in Place 30 sec.	Running in Place 30 sec.	Running in Place 30 sec.
Half Jumping Jacks 25	Half Jumping Jacks 30	Half Jumping Jacks 25	Half Jumping Jacks 30	Half Jumping Jacks 25
60–90 sec. Rest	60–90 sec. Rest	60–90 sec. Rest	60–90 sec. Rest	60–90 sec. Rest
STRETCHES	**STRETCHES**	**LEGS**	**STRETCHES**	**STRETCHES**
Bend Overs	Chest	Walking Lunges 30 yds. (2x)	Chest	Bend Overs
Cross Overs	Lat	High Knees 30 yds. (2x)	Lat	Cross Overs
Inner Thigh	Shoulders	Frog Hops 30 yds. (2x)	Shoulders	Inner Thigh
Forward Lunge	Tricep	Star Hops 12	Tricep	Forward Lunge
Side & Oblique	Partner	Mountain Climbers 12	Partner	Side & Oblique
Hurdler	Arm Rotation	**SPRINTS**	Arm Rotation	Hurdler
Butterfly	60–90 sec. Rest	Intervals (Optional)	60–90 sec. Rest	Butterfly
ITB	**UPPER BODY**	4 Laps = 1600 yds.	**CIRCUIT— UPPER BODY**	ITB
Thigh	Neck Rotations 26			Thigh
Calf	Back Contractions 26		**SET 1**	Calf
60–90 sec. Rest	Swimmer Exercise 14		Regular Pull-Ups 5	60–90 sec. Rest
CIRCUIT— LEGS	Back Lifts 12		Bar Dips 5	**LEGS**
	60–90 sec. Rest		Regular Push-Ups 10	Lunges 21
SET 1	**PULL-UPS**		**SET 2**	Squats 31
The Wall 1:30 min.	Regular 2-4-6-4-2		Close Grip Pull-Ups 5	Fire Hydrants 17 (Each Side)
Frog Hops 30 yds. (2x)	Close Grip 2-4-2		Bar Dips 5	Mountain Climber 13
Hand to Toe 25	Reverse 2-4-2		Diamond Push-Ups 8	The Wall 1:30 sec.
SET 2	Commandos 1-2-1		**SET 3**	60–90 sec. Rest
Walking Lunges 30 yds. (2x)	Behind the Neck 2-4-2		Reverse Grip Pull-Ups 5	**CALVES**
Star Hops 10	60–90 sec. Rest		Bar Dips 5	Straight (Regular) 55
Side Sit-Ups 25	**BAR DIPS**		Dive Bombers 8	Toe to Toe 55
SET 3	Regular 7		**SET 4**	Heel to Heel 55
Mountain Climbers 10	60–90 sec. Rest		Behind the Neck Pull-Ups 3	60–90 sec. Rest
Regular Calf Raises 50	**PUSH-UPS**		Bar Dips 5	**ABDOMINALS**
Knee Bends 25	Regular 2-4-6-8-10-8-6-4-2	**ABDOMINALS**	Regular Push-Ups 10	Hand to Toes 13
SET 4	Diamond 2-4-6-8-6-4-2	Clockwork 20-15-10	Take "After" Supplements	X Sit-Ups 13
Fire Hydrants 25 (Each Side)	Dive Bombers 2-4-6-8-6-4-2	Hanging Knee Up 13	Drink 16 oz. of water	Crunches 13
Toe to Toe Calf Raises 50	8 Count Body Builders 7	Hanging Side Sit-Up 6		Side Sit-Ups 13
Crunches 25	Take "After" Supplements	Hand to Toes (Short) 13		Obliques 13
SET 5	Drink 16 oz. of water	Crunches (Short) 13		Flutter Kicks 13
Heel to Heel Calf Raises 50		Side Sit-Up (Short) 13		Reverse Crunches 13
Knee Roll Ups 25		Obliques (Short) 13		Knee Bends 13
Take "After" Supplements		Atomic 6		Chest Roll 13
Drink 16 oz. of water		Take "After" Supplements		Take "After" Supplements
		Drink 16 oz. of water		Drink 1 quart of water

MONDAY
- MEALS: 1 2 3 4 5
- WATER: 1 2 3 4 5 6 7 8
- SUPPLEMENTS
  - Before: 3 Electrolyte™ / 1 Energy Plus™
  - After: 3 Recover™ / 2 Restore™

TUESDAY
- MEALS: 1 2 3 4 5
- WATER: 1 2 3 4 5 6 7 8
- SUPPLEMENTS
  - Before: 3 Electrolyte™ / 1 Energy Plus™
  - After: 3 Recover™ / 2 Restore™

WEDNESDAY
- MEALS: 1 2 3 4 5
- WATER: 1 2 3 4 5 6 7 8
- SUPPLEMENTS
  - Before: 3 Electrolyte™ / 1 Energy Plus™
  - After: 3 Recover™ / 2 Restore™

THURSDAY
- MEALS: 1 2 3 4 5
- WATER: 1 2 3 4 5 6 7 8
- SUPPLEMENTS
  - Before: 3 Electrolyte™ / 1 Energy Plus™
  - After: 3 Recover™ / 2 Restore™

FRIDAY
- MEALS: 1 2 3 4 5
- WATER: 1 2 3 4 5 6 7 8
- SUPPLEMENTS
  - Before: 3 Electrolyte™ / 1 Energy Plus™
  - After: 3 Recover™ / 2 Restore™

WEEK 6 — BEGINNING LEVEL

✓ MONDAY / /	✓ TUESDAY / /	✓ WEDNESDAY / /	✓ THURSDAY / /	✓ FRIDAY / /
Take "Before" Supplements	Take "Before" Supplements	Take "Before" Supplements	Take "Before" Supplements	Take "Before" Supplements
Drink 16 oz. of water	Drink 16 oz. of water	Drink 16 oz. of water	Drink 16 oz. of water	Drink 16 oz. of water
WARM-UPS	**WARM-UPS**	**WARM-UPS**	**WARM-UPS**	**WARM-UPS**
Jumping Jacks 25	Jumping Jacks 30	Jumping Jacks 25	Jumping Jacks 30	Jumping Jacks 25
Running in Place 30 sec.	Running in Place 30 sec.	Running in Place 30 sec.	Running in Place 30 sec.	Running in Place 30 sec.
Half Jumping Jacks 25	Half Jumping Jacks 30	Half Jumping Jacks 25	Half Jumping Jacks 30	Half Jumping Jacks 25
60–90 sec. Rest	60–90 sec. Rest	60–90 sec. Rest	60–90 sec. Rest	60–90 sec. Rest
STRETCHES	**STRETCHES**	**LEGS**	**STRETCHES**	**STRETCHES**
Bend Overs	Chest	Walking Lunges 20 yds. (3x)	Chest	Bend Overs
Cross Overs	Lat	High Knees 20 yds. (3x)	Lat	Cross Overs
Inner Thigh	Shoulders	Frog Hops 20 yds. (3x)	Shoulders	Inner Thigh
Forward Lunge	Tricep	Star Hops 14	Tricep	Forward Lunge
Side & Oblique	Partner	Mountain Climbers 14	Partner	Side & Oblique
Hurdler	Arm Rotation	**SPRINTS**	Arm Rotation	Hurdler
Butterfly	60–90 sec. Rest	Basic Sprints (Optional)	*TIMED INTERVALS*	Butterfly
ITB	**UPPER BODY**	800 yd. Warm-Up	**UPPER BODY**	ITB
Thigh	Neck Rotations 28	3 Sets of Cones	Neck Rotations 30 sec.	Thigh
Calf	Back Contractions 28	First Set — 50%	Back Contractions 30 sec.	Calf
TIMED INTERVALS	Swimmer Exercise 14	Second Set — 75%	Swimmer Exercise 30 sec.	60–90 sec. Rest
LEGS	Back Lifts 12	Third Set — 100%	Back Lifts 30 sec.	**LEGS**
Lunges 30 sec.	60–90 sec. Rest	7 Sets	60–90 sec. Rest	Lunges 23
Squats 30 sec.	**PULL-UPS**		**PULL-UPS**	Squats 33
Fire Hydrants 30 sec. (Each Side)	Regular 2-4-6-4-2		Regular 30 sec.	Fire Hydrants 19 (Each Side)
Mountain Climber 30 sec.	Close Grip 2-4-2		Close Grip 30 sec.	Mountain Climber 14
The Wall 1:30 min.	Reverse 2-4-2		Reverse 30 sec.	The Wall 1:30 min.
60–90 sec. Rest	Commandos 1-2-1		Commandos 30 sec.	60–90 sec. Rest
CALVES	Behind the Neck 2-4-2		Behind the Neck 30 sec.	**CALVES**
Straight (Regular) 30 sec.	60–90 sec. Rest		60–90 sec. Rest	Straight (Regular) 60
Toe to Toe 30 sec.	**BAR DIPS**		**BAR DIPS**	Toe to Toe 60
Heel to Heel 30 sec.	Regular 7		Regular 30 sec.	Heel to Heel 60
60–90 sec. Rest	60–90 sec. Rest		60–90 sec. Rest	60–90 sec. Rest
ABDOMINALS	**PUSH-UPS**		**PUSH-UPS**	**ABDOMINALS**
Hand to Toes 30 sec.	Regular 2-4-6-8-10-8-6-4-2	**ABDOMINALS**	Regular 30 sec.	Hand to Toes 15
X Sit-Ups 30 sec.	Diamond 2-4-6-8-6-4-2	Clockwork 20-15-10	Diamond 30 sec.	X Sit-Ups 15
Crunches 30 sec.	Dive Bombers 2-4-6-8-6-4-2	Hanging Knee Up 15	Dive Bombers 30 sec.	Crunches 15
Side Sit-Ups 30 sec.	8 Count Body Builders 7	Hanging Side Sit-Up 7	8 Count Body Builders 30 sec.	Side Sit-Ups 15
Obliques 30 sec.	Take "After" Supplements	Hand to Toes (Short) 15	Take "After" Supplements	Obliques 15
Flutter Kicks 30 sec.	Drink 16 oz. of water	Crunches (Short) 15	Drink 16 oz. of water	Flutter Kicks 15
Reverse Crunches 30 sec.		Side Sit-Up (Short) 15		Reverse Crunches 15
Knee Bends 30 sec.		Obliques (Short) 15		Knee Bends 15
Chest Roll 30 sec.		Atomic 8		Chest Roll 15
Take "After" Supplements		Take "After" Supplements		Take "After" Supplements
Drink 16 oz. of water		Drink 16 oz. of water		Drink 1 quart of water

	MONDAY	TUESDAY	WEDNESDAY	THURSDAY	FRIDAY
MEALS	1 2 3 4 5	1 2 3 4 5	1 2 3 4 5	1 2 3 4 5	1 2 3 4 5
WATER	1 2 3 4 5 6 7 8	1 2 3 4 5 6 7 8	1 2 3 4 5 6 7 8	1 2 3 4 5 6 7 8	1 2 3 4 5 6 7 8

SUPPLEMENTS

	Before	After
MONDAY	3 Electrolyte™ / 1 Energy Plus™	3 Recover™ / 2 Restore™
TUESDAY	3 Electrolyte™ / 1 Energy Plus™	3 Recover™ / 2 Restore™
WEDNESDAY	3 Electrolyte™ / 1 Energy Plus™	3 Recover™ / 2 Restore™
THURSDAY	3 Electrolyte™ / 1 Energy Plus™	3 Recover™ / 2 Restore™
FRIDAY	3 Electrolyte™ / 1 Energy Plus™	3 Recover™ / 2 Restore™

WEEK 7 — BEGINNING LEVEL

✓ MONDAY / /	✓ TUESDAY / /	✓ WEDNESDAY / /	✓ THURSDAY / /	✓ FRIDAY / /
Take "Before" Supplements	Take "Before" Supplements	Take "Before" Supplements	Take "Before" Supplements	Take "Before" Supplements
Drink 16 oz. of water	Drink 16 oz. of water	Drink 16 oz. of water	Drink 16 oz. of water	Drink 16 oz. of water
WARM-UPS	**WARM-UPS**	**WARM-UPS**	**WARM-UPS**	**WARM-UPS**
Jumping Jacks 25	Jumping Jacks 30	Jumping Jacks 25	Jumping Jacks 30	Jumping Jacks 25
Running in Place 30 sec.	Running in Place 30 sec.	Running in Place 30 sec.	Running in Place 30 sec.	Running in Place 30 sec.
Half Jumping Jacks 25	Half Jumping Jacks 30	Half Jumping Jacks 25	Half Jumping Jacks 30	Half Jumping Jacks 25
60–90 sec. Rest	60–90 sec. Rest	60–90 sec. Rest	60–90 sec. Rest	60–90 sec. Rest
STRETCHES	**STRETCHES**	**LEGS**	**STRETCHES**	**STRETCHES**
Bend Overs	Chest	Walking Lunges 25 yds. (3x)	Chest	Bend Overs
Cross Overs	Lat	High Knees 25 yds. (3x)	Lat	Cross Overs
Inner Thigh	Shoulders	Frog Hops 25 yds. (3x)	Shoulders	Inner Thigh
Forward Lunge	Tricep	Star Hops 15	Tricep	Forward Lunge
Side & Oblique	Partner	Mountain Climbers 15	Partner	Side & Oblique
Hurdler	Arm Rotation	**SPRINTS**	Arm Rotation	Hurdler
Butterfly	60–90 sec. Rest	Intervals (Optional)	60–90 sec. Rest	Butterfly
ITB	**UPPER BODY**	5 Laps = 2000 yds.	**UPPER BODY**	ITB
Thigh	Neck Rotations 16		Neck Rotations 16	Thigh
Calf	Back Contractions 16		Back Contractions 16	Calf
60–90 sec. Rest	Swimmer Exercise 16		Swimmer Exercise 16	60–90 sec. Rest
LEGS	Back Lifts 13		Back Lifts 13	**LEGS**
Lunges 25	60–90 sec. Rest		60–90 sec. Rest	Lunges 25
Squats 35	**PULL-UPS**		**PULL-UPS**	Squats 35
Fire Hydrants 21 (Each Side)	Regular 2-4-6-8-6-4-2		Regular 2-4-6-8-6-4-2	Fire Hydrants 21 (Each Side)
Mountain Climber 15	Close Grip 2-4-6-4-2		Close Grip 2-4-6-4-2	Mountain Climber 15
The Wall 1:30 min.	Reverse 2-4-6-4-2		Reverse 2-4-6-4-2	The Wall 1:30 sec.
60–90 sec. Rest	Commandos 2-4-2		Commandos 2-4-2	60–90 sec. Rest
CALVES	Behind the Neck 1-2-3-4-5		Behind the Neck 1-2-3-4-5	**CALVES**
Straight (Regular) 60	60–90 sec. Rest		60–90 sec. Rest	Straight (Regular) 60
Toe to Toe 60	**BAR DIPS**		**BAR DIPS**	Toe to Toe 60
Heel to Heel 60	Regular 8		Regular 8	Heel to Heel 60
60–90 sec. Rest	60–90 sec. Rest		60–90 sec. Rest	60–90 sec. Rest
ABDOMINALS	**PUSH-UPS**	**ABDOMINALS**	**PUSH-UPS**	**ABDOMINALS**
Hand to Toes 17	Regular 2-4-6-8-10-8-6-4-2	Clockwork 20-15-10	Regular 2-4-6-8-10-8-6-4-2	Hand to Toes 17
X Sit-Ups 17	Diamond 2-4-6-4-2	Hanging Knee Up 17	Diamond 2-4-6-4-2	X Sit-Ups 17
Crunches 17	Dive Bombers 2-4-6-4-2	Hanging Side Sit-Up 8	Dive Bombers 2-4-6-4-2	Crunches 17
Side Sit-Ups 17	8 Count Body Builders 8	Hand to Toes (Short) 17	8 Count Body Builders 8	Side Sit-Ups 17
Obliques 17	Take "After" Supplements	Crunches (Short) 17	Take "After" Supplements	Obliques 17
Flutter Kicks 17	Drink 16 oz. of water	Side Sit-Up (Short) 17	Drink 16 oz. of water	Flutter Kicks 17
Reverse Crunches 17		Obliques (Short) 17		Reverse Crunches 17
Knee Bends 17		Atomic 10		Knee Bends 17
Chest Roll 17		Take "After" Supplements		Chest Roll 17
Take "After" Supplements		Drink 16 oz. of water		Take "After" Supplements
Drink 16 oz. of water				Drink 1 quart of water

MEALS / WATER / SUPPLEMENTS (each day)

MEALS: 1 2 3 4 5
WATER: 1 2 3 4 5 6 7 8

SUPPLEMENTS

Before	After
3 Electrolyte™	3 Recover™
1 Energy Plus™	2 Restore™

(repeated for Monday, Tuesday, Wednesday, Thursday, Friday)

WEEK 8   BEGINNING LEVEL

✓ **MONDAY** / /	✓ **TUESDAY** / /	✓ **WEDNESDAY** / /	✓ **THURSDAY** / /	✓ **FRIDAY** / /
Take "Before" Supplements	Take "Before" Supplements	Take "Before" Supplements	Take "Before" Supplements	Take "Before" Supplements
Drink 16 oz. of water	Drink 16 oz. of water	Drink 16 oz. of water	Drink 16 oz. of water	Drink 16 oz. of water
WARM-UPS	**WARM-UPS**	**WARM-UPS**	**WARM-UPS**	**WARM-UPS**
Jumping Jacks 25	Jumping Jacks 30	Jumping Jacks 25	Jumping Jacks 30	Jumping Jacks 25
Running in Place 30 sec.	Running in Place 30 sec.	Running in Place 30 sec.	Running in Place 30 sec.	Running in Place 30 sec.
Half Jumping Jacks 25	Half Jumping Jacks 30	Half Jumping Jacks 25	Half Jumping Jacks 30	Half Jumping Jacks 25
60–90 sec. Rest	60–90 sec. Rest	60–90 sec. Rest	60–90 sec. Rest	60–90 sec. Rest
STRETCHES	**STRETCHES**	**LEGS**	**STRETCHES**	**STRETCHES**
Bend Overs	Chest	Walking Lunges 30 yds. (3x)	Chest	Bend Overs
Cross Overs	Lat	High Knees 30 yds. (3x)	Lat	Cross Overs
Inner Thigh	Shoulders	Frog Hops 30 yds. (3x)	Shoulders	Inner Thigh
Forward Lunge	Tricep	Star Hops 15	Tricep	Forward Lunge
Side & Oblique	Partner	Mountain Climbers 15	Partner	Side & Oblique
Hurdler	Arm Rotation	**SPRINTS**	Arm Rotation	Hurdler
Butterfly	60–90 sec. Rest	Basic Sprints (Optional)	60–90 sec. Rest	Butterfly
ITB	**UPPER BODY**	3 Sets of Cones	**UPPER BODY**	ITB
Thigh	Neck Rotations 16	First Set — 50%	Neck Rotations 16	Thigh
Calf	Back Contractions 16	Second Set — 75%	Back Contractions 16	Calf
60–90 sec. Rest	Swimmer Exercise 16	Third Set — 100%	Swimmer Exercise 16	60–90 sec. Rest
LEGS	Back Lifts 13	8 Sets	Back Lifts 13	**LEGS**
Lunges 27	60–90 sec. Rest		60–90 sec. Rest	Lunges 27
Squats 37	**PULL-UPS**		**PULL-UPS**	Squats 37
Fire Hydrants 21 (Each Side)	Regular 2-4-6-8-6-4-2		Regular 2-4-6-8-6-4-2	Fire Hydrants 21 (Each Side)
Mountain Climber 16	Close Grip 2-4-6-4-2		Close Grip 2-4-6-4-2	Mountain Climber 16
The Wall 1:30 min.	Reverse 2-4-6-4-2		Reverse 2-4-6-4-2	The Wall 1:30 min.
60–90 sec. Rest	Commandos 2-4-2		Commandos 2-4-2	60–90 sec. Rest
CALVES	Behind the Neck 1-3-5-3-1		Behind the Neck 1-3-5-3-1	**CALVES**
Straight (Regular) 65	60–90 sec. Rest		60–90 sec. Rest	Straight (Regular) 65
Toe to Toe 65	**BAR DIPS**		**BAR DIPS**	Toe to Toe 65
Heel to Heel 65	Regular 8		Regular 8	Heel to Heel 65
60–90 sec. Rest	60–90 sec. Rest		60–90 sec. Rest	60–90 sec. Rest
ABDOMINALS	**PUSH-UPS**	**ABDOMINALS**	**PUSH-UPS**	**ABDOMINALS**
Hand to Toes 19	Regular 2-4-6-8-10-8-6-4-2	Clockwork 20-15-10	Regular 2-4-6-8-10-8-6-4-2	Hand to Toes 19
X Sit-Ups 19	Diamond 1-3-5-7-9-11 ⬇	Hanging Knee Up 19	Diamond 1-3-5-7-9-11 ⬇	X Sit-Ups 19
Crunches 19	Dive Bombers 1-3-5-7-9-11 ⬇	Hanging Side Sit-Up 9	Dive Bombers 1-3-5-7-9-11 ⬇	Crunches 19
Side Sit-Ups 19	8 Count Body Builders 8	Hand to Toes (Short) 19	8 Count Body Builders 8	Side Sit-Ups 19
Obliques 19	Take "After" Supplements	Crunches (Short) 19	Take "After" Supplements	Obliques 19
Flutter Kicks 19	Drink 16 oz. of water	Side Sit-Up (Short) 19	Drink 16 oz. of water	Flutter Kicks 19
Reverse Crunches 19		Obliques (Short) 19		Reverse Crunches 19
Knee Bends 19		Atomic 12		Knee Bends 19
Chest Roll 19		Take "After" Supplements		Chest Roll 19
Take "After" Supplements		Drink 16 oz. of water		Take "After" Supplements
Drink 16 oz. of water				Drink 1 quart of water

MEALS	**WATER**	**MEALS**	**WATER**	**MEALS**	**WATER**	**MEALS**	**WATER**	**MEALS**	**WATER**
1 2 3 4 5	1 2 3 4 5 6 7 8	1 2 3 4 5	1 2 3 4 5 6 7 8	1 2 3 4 5	1 2 3 4 5 6 7 8	1 2 3 4 5	1 2 3 4 5 6 7 8	1 2 3 4 5	1 2 3 4 5 6 7 8

SUPPLEMENTS	**SUPPLEMENTS**	**SUPPLEMENTS**	**SUPPLEMENTS**	**SUPPLEMENTS**
Before 3 Electrolyte™ / 1 Energy Plus™ **After** 3 Recover™ / 2 Restore™	**Before** 3 Electrolyte™ / 1 Energy Plus™ **After** 3 Recover™ / 2 Restore™	**Before** 3 Electrolyte™ / 1 Energy Plus™ **After** 3 Recover™ / 2 Restore™	**Before** 3 Electrolyte™ / 1 Energy Plus™ **After** 3 Recover™ / 2 Restore™	**Before** 3 Electrolyte™ / 1 Energy Plus™ **After** 3 Recover™ / 2 Restore™

✓ **MONDAY** / /	✓ **TUESDAY** / /	✓ **WEDNESDAY** / /	✓ **THURSDAY** / /	✓ **FRIDAY** / /
Take "Before" Supplements	Take "Before" Supplements	Take "Before" Supplements	Take "Before" Supplements	Take "Before" Supplements
Drink 16 oz. of water	Drink 16 oz. of water	Drink 16 oz. of water	Drink 16 oz. of water	Drink 16 oz. of water
WARM-UPS	**WARM-UPS**	**WARM-UPS**	**WARM-UPS**	**WARM-UPS**
Jumping Jacks 25	Jumping Jacks 30	Jumping Jacks 25	Jumping Jacks 30	Jumping Jacks 25
Running in Place 30 sec.	Running in Place 30 sec.	Running in Place 30 sec.	Running in Place 30 sec.	Running in Place 30 sec.
Half Jumping Jacks 25	Half Jumping Jacks 30	Half Jumping Jacks 25	Half Jumping Jacks 30	Half Jumping Jacks 25
60–90 sec. Rest	60–90 sec. Rest	60–90 sec. Rest	60–90 sec. Rest	60–90 sec. Rest
STRETCHES	**STRETCHES**	**LEGS**	**STRETCHES**	**STRETCHES**
Bend Overs	Chest	Walking Lunges 30 yds. (3x)	Chest	Bend Overs
Cross Overs	Lat	High Knees 30 yds. (3x)	Lat	Cross Overs
Inner Thigh	Shoulders	Frog Hops 30 yds. (3x)	Shoulders	Inner Thigh
Forward Lunge	Tricep	Star Hops 15	Tricep	Forward Lunge
Side & Oblique	Partner	Mountain Climbers 15	Partner	Side & Oblique
Hurdler	Arm Rotation	**SPRINTS**	Arm Rotation	Hurdler
Butterfly	60–90 sec. Rest	Intervals (Optional)	60–90 sec. Rest	Butterfly
ITB	**UPPER BODY**	6 Laps = 2400 yds.	**BURNOUTS— UPPER BODY**	ITB
Thigh	Neck Rotations 18			Thigh
Calf	Back Contractions 18		**SET 1**	Calf
60–90 sec. Rest	Swimmer Exercise 18		Regular Pull-Ups	60–90 sec. Rest
BURNOUTS— LEGS	Back Lifts 14		Bar Dips	**LEGS**
	60–90 sec. Rest		Regular Push-Ups	Lunges 29
SET 1	**PULL-UPS**		**SET 2**	Squats 39
The Wall	Regular 2-4-6-8-6-4-2		Close Grip Pull-Ups	Fire Hydrants 23 (Each Side)
Frog Hops	Close Grip 2-4-6-4-2		Bar Dips	Mountain Climber 17
Hand to Toe	Reverse 2-4-6-4-2		Diamond Push-Ups	The Wall 1:45 min.
SET 2	Commandos 2-4-2		**SET 3**	60–90 sec. Rest
Lunges	Behind the Neck 1-3-5-3-1		Reverse Grip Pull-Ups	**CALVES**
Star Hops	60–90 sec. Rest		Bar Dips	Straight (Regular) 65
Side Sit-Ups	**BAR DIPS**		Dive Bombers	Toe to Toe 65
SET 3	Regular 9		**SET 4**	Heel to Heel 65
Mountain Climbers	60–90 sec. Rest		Behind the Neck Pull-Ups	60–90 sec. Rest
Knee Bends	**PUSH-UPS**		Bar Dips	**ABDOMINALS**
SET 4	Reg. 2-4-6-8-10-12-10-8-6-4-2	**ABDOMINALS**	Regular Push-Ups	Hand to Toes 21
Fire Hydrants (Each Side)	Diamond 1-3-5-7-9-11 ↓	Clockwork 25-20-15	**SET 5**	X Sit-Ups 21
High Knees	Dive Bombers 1-3-5-7-9-11 ↓	Hanging Knee Up 21	Commandos	Crunches 21
Crunches	8 Count Body Builders 9	Hanging Side Sit-Up 10	Bar Dips	Side Sit-Ups 21
SET 5	Take "After" Supplements	Hand to Toe (Short) 21	Diamond Push-Ups	Obliques 21
Calf Raises	Drink 16 oz. of water	Crunches (Short) 21	Take "After" Supplements	Flutter Kicks 21
Sprints		Side Sit-Up (Short) 21	Drink 16 oz. of water	Reverse Crunches 21
Knee Roll Ups		Obliques (Short) 21		Knee Bends 21
Take "After" Supplements		Atomic 14		Chest Roll 21
Drink 16 oz. of water		Take "After" Supplements		Take "After" Supplements
		Drink 16 oz. of water		Drink 1 quart of water

MEALS	WATER	MEALS	WATER	MEALS	WATER	MEALS	WATER	MEALS	WATER
1 2 3 4 5	1 2 3 4 5 6 7 8	1 2 3 4 5	1 2 3 4 5 6 7 8	1 2 3 4 5	1 2 3 4 5 6 7 8	1 2 3 4 5	1 2 3 4 5 6 7 8	1 2 3 4 5	1 2 3 4 5 6 7 8

SUPPLEMENTS

Before	After	Before	After	Before	After	Before	After	Before	After
3 Electrolyte™	**3** Recover™	**3** Electrolyte™	**3** Recover™	**3** Electrolyte™	**3** Recover™	**3** Electrolyte™	**3** Recover™	**3** Electrolyte™	**3** Recover™
1 Energy Plus™	**2** Restore™	**1** Energy Plus™	**2** Restore™	**1** Energy Plus™	**2** Restore™	**1** Energy Plus™	**2** Restore™	**1** Energy Plus™	**2** Restore™

WEEK 10 — BEGINNING LEVEL

✓ MONDAY / /	✓ TUESDAY / /	✓ WEDNESDAY / /	✓ THURSDAY / /	✓ FRIDAY / /
Take "Before" Supplements	Take "Before" Supplements	Take "Before" Supplements	Take "Before" Supplements	Take "Before" Supplements
Drink 16 oz. of water	Drink 16 oz. of water	Drink 16 oz. of water	Drink 16 oz. of water	Drink 16 oz. of water
WARM-UPS	**WARM-UPS**	**WARM-UPS**	**WARM-UPS**	**WARM-UPS**
Jumping Jacks 25	Jumping Jacks 30	Jumping Jacks 25	Jumping Jacks 30	Jumping Jacks 25
Running in Place 30 sec.	Running in Place 30 sec.	Running in Place 30 sec.	Running in Place 30 sec.	Running in Place 30 sec.
Half Jumping Jacks 25	Half Jumping Jacks 30	Half Jumping Jacks 325	Half Jumping Jacks 30	Half Jumping Jacks 25
60–90 sec. Rest	60–90 sec. Rest	60–90 sec. Rest	60–90 sec. Rest	60–90 sec. Rest
STRETCHES	**STRETCHES**	**LEGS**	**STRETCHES**	**STRETCHES**
Bend Overs	Chest	Walking Lunges 30 yds. (3x)	Chest	Bend Overs
Cross Overs	Lat	High Knees 30 yds. (3x)	Lat	Cross Overs
Inner Thigh	Shoulders	Frog Hops 30 yds. (3x)	Shoulders	Inner Thigh
Forward Lunge	Tricep	Star Hops 15	Tricep	Forward Lunge
Side & Oblique	Partner	Mountain Climbers 15	Partner	Side & Oblique
Hurdler	Arm Rotation	**SPRINTS**	Arm Rotation	Hurdler
Butterfly	60–90 sec. Rest	Basic Sprints (Optional)	60–90 sec. Rest	Butterfly
ITB	**UPPER BODY**	3 Sets of Cones	**UPPER BODY**	ITB
Thigh	Neck Rotations 18	First Set — 50%	Neck Rotations 18	Thigh
Calf	Back Contractions 18	Second Set — 75%	Back Contractions 18	Calf
60–90 sec. Rest	Swimmer Exercise 18	Third Set — 100%	Swimmer Exercise 18	60–90 sec. Rest
LEGS	Back Lifts 14	9 Sets	Back Lifts 14	**LEGS**
Lunges 31	60–90 sec. Rest		60–90 sec. Rest	Lunges 31
Squats 41	**PULL-UPS**		**PULL-UPS**	Squats 41
Fire Hydrants 23 (Each Side)	Regular 2-4-6-8-10-8-6-4-2		Regular 2-4-6-8-10-8-6-4-2	Fire Hydrants 23 (Each Side)
Mountain Climber 18	Close Grip 2-4-6-8-6-4-2		Close Grip 2-4-6-8-6-4-2	Mountain Climber 18
The Wall 1:45 min.	Reverse 2-4-6-8-6-4-2		Reverse 2-4-6-8-6-4-2	The Wall 1:45 min.
60–90 sec. Rest	Commandos 2-4-6-4-2		Commandos 2-4-6-4-2	60–90 sec. Rest
CALVES	Behind the Neck 2-4-6-4-2		Behind the Neck 2-4-6-4-2	**CALVES**
Straight (Regular) 70	60–90 sec. Rest		60–90 sec. Rest	Straight (Regular) 70
Toe to Toe 70	**BAR DIPS**		**BAR DIPS**	Toe to Toe 70
Heel to Heel 70	Regular 9		Regular 9	Heel to Heel 70
60–90 sec. Rest	60–90 sec. Rest		60–90 sec. Rest	60–90 sec. Rest
ABDOMINALS	**PUSH-UPS**	**ABDOMINALS**	**PUSH-UPS**	**ABDOMINALS**
Hand to Toes 23	Reg. 2-4-6-8-10-12 ⬇	Clockwork 25-20-15	Reg. 2-4-6-8-10-12 ⬇	Hand to Toes 23
X Sit-Ups 23	Diamond 2-4-6-8-10-12 ⬇	Hanging Knee Up 23	Diamond 1-3-5-7-9-11 ⬇	X Sit-Ups 23
Crunches 23	Dive Bombers 2-4-6-8-10-12 ⬇	Hanging Side Sit-Up 11	Dive Bombers 2-4-6-8-10-12 ⬇	Crunches 23
Side Sit-Ups 23	8 Count Body Builders 9	Hand to Toe (Short) 23	8 Count Body Builders 9	Side Sit-Ups 23
Obliques 23	Take "After" Supplements	Crunches (Short) 23	Take "After" Supplements	Obliques 23
Flutter Kicks 23	Drink 16 oz. of water	Side Sit-Up (Short) 23	Drink 16 oz. of water	Flutter Kicks 23
Reverse Crunches 23		Obliques (Short) 23		Reverse Crunches 23
Knee Bends 23		Atomic 16		Knee Bends 23
Chest Roll 23		Take "After" Supplements		Chest Roll 23
Take "After" Supplements		Drink 16 oz. of water		Take "After" Supplements
Drink 16 oz. of water				Drink 1 quart of water

MONDAY / /

- ✓ Take "Before" Supplements
- Drink 16 oz. of water

WARM-UPS
- Jumping Jacks 25
- Running in Place 30 sec.
- Half Jumping Jacks 25
- 60–90 sec. Rest

STRETCHES
- Bend Overs
- Cross Overs
- Inner Thigh
- Forward Lunge
- Side & Oblique
- Hurdler
- Butterfly
- ITB
- Thigh
- Calf
- 60–90 sec. Rest

CIRCUIT—LEGS
SET 1
- The Wall 2:00 min.
- Frog Hops 30 yds. (3x)
- Hand to Toe 25

SET 2
- Walking Lunges 30 yds. (3x)
- Star Hops 10
- Side Sit-Ups 25

SET 3
- Mountain Climbers 10
- Regular Calf Raises 50
- Knee Bends 25

SET 4
- Fire Hydrants 25 (Each Side)
- Toe to Toe Calf Raises 50
- Crunches 25

SET 5
- Heel to Heel Calf Raises 50
- Knee Roll Ups 25
- Take "After" Supplements
- Drink 16 oz. of water

TUESDAY / /

- ✓ Take "Before" Supplements
- Drink 16 oz. of water

WARM-UPS
- Jumping Jacks 30
- Running in Place 30 sec.
- Half Jumping Jacks 30
- 60–90 sec. Rest

STRETCHES
- Chest
- Lat
- Shoulders
- Tricep
- Partner
- Arm Rotation
- 60–90 sec. Rest

CIRCUIT—UPPER BODY
SET 1
- Regular Pull-Ups 7
- Bar Dips 7
- Regular Push-Ups 15

SET 2
- Close Grip Pull-Ups 7
- Bar Dips 7
- Diamond Push-Ups 10

SET 3
- Reverse Grip Pull-Ups 7
- Bar Dips 7
- Dive Bombers 10

SET 4
- Behind the Neck Pull-Ups 5
- Bar Dips 7
- Regular Push-Ups 15
- Take "After" Supplements
- Drink 16 oz. of water

WEDNESDAY / /

- ✓ Take "Before" Supplements
- Drink 16 oz. of water

WARM-UPS
- Jumping Jacks 25
- Running in Place 30 sec.
- Half Jumping Jacks 25
- 60–90 sec. Rest

LEGS
- Walking Lunges 30 yds. (3x)
- High Knees 30 yds. (3x)
- Frog Hops 30 yds. (3x)
- Star Hops 15
- Mountain Climbers 15

SPRINTS
- Intervals (Optional)
- 6 Laps = 2400 yds.

ABDOMINALS
- Clockwork 25-20-15
- Hanging Knee Up 25
- Hanging Side Sit-Up 12
- Hand to Toe (Short) 25
- Crunches (Short) 25
- Side Sit-Up (Short) 25
- Obliques (Short) 25
- Atomic 18
- Take "After" Supplements
- Drink 16 oz. of water

THURSDAY / /

- ✓ Take "Before" Supplements
- Drink 16 oz. of water

WARM-UPS
- Jumping Jacks 30
- Running in Place 30 sec.
- Half Jumping Jacks 30
- 60–90 sec. Rest

STRETCHES
- Chest
- Lat
- Shoulders
- Tricep
- Partner
- Arm Rotation

TIMED INTERVALS — UPPER BODY
- Neck Rotations 45 sec.
- Back Contractions 45 sec.
- Swimmer Exercise 45 sec.
- Back Lifts 45 sec.
- 60–90 sec. Rest

PULL-UPS
- Regular 45 sec.
- Close Grip 45 sec.
- Reverse 45 sec.
- Commandos 45 sec.
- Behind the Neck 45 sec.
- 60–90 sec. Rest

BAR DIPS
- Regular 45 sec.
- 60–90 sec. Rest

PUSH-UPS
- Regular 45 sec.
- Diamond 45 sec.
- Dive Bombers 45 sec.
- 8 Count Body Builders 45 sec.
- Take "After" Supplements
- Drink 16 oz. of water

FRIDAY / /

- ✓ Take "Before" Supplements
- Drink 16 oz. of water

WARM-UPS
- Jumping Jacks 25
- Running in Place 30 sec.
- Half Jumping Jacks 25
- 60–90 sec. Rest

STRETCHES
- Bend Overs
- Cross Overs
- Inner Thigh
- Forward Lunge
- Side & Oblique
- Hurdler
- Butterfly
- ITB
- Thigh
- Calf

TIMED INTERVALS — LEGS
- Lunges 45 sec.
- Squats 45 sec.
- Fire Hydrants 45 sec. (Each Side)
- Mountain Climber 45 sec.
- The Wall 2:00 min.
- 60–90 sec. Rest

CALVES
- Straight (Regular) 45 sec.
- Toe to Toe 45 sec.
- Heel to Heel 45 sec.
- 60–90 sec. Rest

ABDOMINALS
- Hand to Toes 45 sec.
- X Sit-Ups 45 sec.
- Crunches 45 sec.
- Side Sit-Ups 45 sec.
- Obliques 45 sec.
- Flutter Kicks 45 sec.
- Reverse Crunches 45 sec.
- Knee Bends 45 sec.
- Chest Roll 45 sec.
- Take "After" Supplements
- Drink 1 quart of water

Daily Tracking (each day: Monday–Friday)

MEALS: 1 2 3 4 5

WATER: 1 2 3 4 5 6 7 8

SUPPLEMENTS

Before	After
3 Electrolyte™	3 Recover™
1 Energy Plus™	2 Restore™

WEEK 12 — BEGINNING LEVEL

✓ MONDAY / /	✓ TUESDAY / /	✓ WEDNESDAY / /	✓ THURSDAY / /	✓ FRIDAY / /
Take "Before" Supplements	Take "Before" Supplements	Take "Before" Supplements	Take "Before" Supplements	Take "Before" Supplements
Drink 16 oz. of water	Drink 16 oz. of water	Drink 16 oz. of water	Drink 16 oz. of water	Drink 16 oz. of water
WARM-UPS	**WARM-UPS**	**WARM-UPS**	**WARM-UPS**	**WARM-UPS**
Jumping Jacks 25	Jumping Jacks 30	Jumping Jacks 25	Jumping Jacks 30	Jumping Jacks 25
Running in Place 30 sec.	Running in Place 30 sec.	Running in Place 30 sec.	Running in Place 30 sec.	Running in Place 30 sec.
Half Jumping Jacks 25	Half Jumping Jacks 30	Half Jumping Jacks 25	Half Jumping Jacks 30	Half Jumping Jacks 25
60–90 sec. Rest	60–90 sec. Rest	60–90 sec. Rest	60–90 sec. Rest	60–90 sec. Rest
STRETCHES	**STRETCHES**	**LEGS**	**STRETCHES**	**STRETCHES**
Bend Overs	Chest	Walking Lunges 30 yds. (3x)	Chest	Bend Overs
Cross Overs	Lat	High Knees 30 yds. (3x)	Lat	Cross Overs
Inner Thigh	Shoulders	Frog Hops 30 yds. (3x)	Shoulders	Inner Thigh
Forward Lunge	Tricep	Star Hops 15	Tricep	Forward Lunge
Side & Oblique	Partner	Mountain Climbers 15	Partner	Side & Oblique
Hurdler	Arm Rotation	**SPRINTS**	Arm Rotation	Hurdler
Butterfly	60–90 sec. Rest	Basic Sprints (Optional)	60–90 sec. Rest	Butterfly
ITB	**UPPER BODY**	3 Sets of Cones	**UPPER BODY**	ITB
Thigh	Neck Rotations 20	First Set — 50%	Neck Rotations 20	Thigh
Calf	Back Contractions 20	Second Set — 75%	Back Contractions 20	Calf
60–90 sec. Rest	Swimmer Exercise 20	Third Set — 100%	Swimmer Exercise 20	60–90 sec. Rest
LEGS	Back Lifts 15	10 Sets	Back Lifts 15	**LEGS**
Lunges 35	60–90 sec. Rest		60–90 sec. Rest	Lunges 35
Squats 45	**PULL-UPS**		**PULL-UPS**	Squats 45
Fire Hydrants 25 (Each Side)	Regular 2-4-6-8-10-8-6-4-2		Regular 2-4-6-8-10-8-6-4-2	Fire Hydrants 25 (Each Side)
Mountain Climber 20	Close Grip 2-4-6-8-6-4-2		Close Grip 2-4-6-8-6-4-2	Mountain Climber 20
The Wall 2:00 min.	Reverse 2-4-6-8-6-4-2		Reverse 2-4-6-8-6-4-2	The Wall 2:00 min.
60–90 sec. Rest	Commandos 2-4-6-4-2		Commandos 2-4-6-4-2	60–90 sec. Rest
CALVES	Behind the Neck 2-4-6-4-2		Behind the Neck 2-4-6-4-2	**CALVES**
Straight (Regular) 75	60–90 sec. Rest		60–90 sec. Rest	Straight (Regular) 75
Toe to Toe 75	**BAR DIPS**		**BAR DIPS**	Toe to Toe 75
Heel to Heel 75	Regular 10		Regular 10	Heel to Heel 75
60–90 sec. Rest	60–90 sec. Rest		60–90 sec. Rest	60–90 sec. Rest
ABDOMINALS	**PUSH-UPS**	**ABDOMINALS**	**PUSH-UPS**	**ABDOMINALS**
Hand to Toes 25	Reg. 2-4-6-8-10-12 ⬇	Clockwork 25-20-15	Reg. 2-4-6-8-10-12 ⬇	Hand to Toes 25
X Sit-Ups 25	Diamond 2-4-6-8-10 ⬇	Hanging Knee Up 25	Diamond 2-4-6-8-10 ⬇	X Sit-Ups 25
Crunches 25	Dive Bombers 2-4-6-8-10 ⬇	Hanging Side Sit-Up 12	Dive Bombers 2-4-6-8-10 ⬇	Crunches 25
Side Sit-Ups 25	8 Count Body Builders 10	Hand to Toe (Short) 25	8 Count Body Builders 10	Side Sit-Ups 25
Obliques 25	Take "After" Supplements	Crunches (Short) 25	Take "After" Supplements	Obliques 25
Flutter Kicks 25	Drink 16 oz. of water	Side Sit-Up (Short) 25	Drink 16 oz. of water	Flutter Kicks 25
Reverse Crunches 25		Obliques (Short) 25		Reverse Crunches 25
Knee Bends 25		Atomic 20		Knee Bends 25
Chest Roll 25		Take "After" Supplements		Chest Roll 25
Take "After" Supplements		Drink 16 oz. of water		Take "After" Supplements
Drink 16 oz. of water				Drink 1 quart of water

MONDAY	TUESDAY	WEDNESDAY	THURSDAY	FRIDAY
MEALS 1 2 3 4 / 5 **WATER** 1 2 3 4 / 5 6 7 8	**MEALS** 1 2 3 4 / 5 **WATER** 1 2 3 4 / 5 6 7 8	**MEALS** 1 2 3 4 / 5 **WATER** 1 2 3 4 / 5 6 7 8	**MEALS** 1 2 3 4 / 5 **WATER** 1 2 3 4 / 5 6 7 8	**MEALS** 1 2 3 4 / 5 **WATER** 1 2 3 4 / 5 6 7 8
SUPPLEMENTS	**SUPPLEMENTS**	**SUPPLEMENTS**	**SUPPLEMENTS**	**SUPPLEMENTS**
Before: 3 Electrolyte™, 1 Energy Plus™ / After: 3 Recover™, 2 Restore™	Before: 3 Electrolyte™, 1 Energy Plus™ / After: 3 Recover™, 2 Restore™	Before: 3 Electrolyte™, 1 Energy Plus™ / After: 3 Recover™, 2 Restore™	Before: 3 Electrolyte™, 1 Energy Plus™ / After: 3 Recover™, 2 Restore™	Before: 3 Electrolyte™, 1 Energy Plus™ / After: 3 Recover™, 2 Restore™

✓ MONDAY / /	✓ TUESDAY / /	✓ WEDNESDAY / /	✓ THURSDAY / /	✓ FRIDAY / /
Take "Before" Supplements	Take "Before" Supplements	Take "Before" Supplements	Take "Before" Supplements	Take "Before" Supplements
Drink 16 oz. of water	Drink 16 oz. of water	Drink 16 oz. of water	Drink 16 oz. of water	Drink 16 oz. of water
WARM-UPS	**WARM-UPS**	**WARM-UPS**	**WARM-UPS**	**WARM-UPS**
Jumping Jacks 35	Jumping Jacks 35	Jumping Jacks 35	Jumping Jacks 35	Jumping Jacks 35
Running in Place 60 sec.	Running in Place 60 sec.	Running in Place 60 sec.	Running in Place 60 sec.	Running in Place 60 sec.
Half Jumping Jacks 35	Half Jumping Jacks 35	Half Jumping Jacks 35	Half Jumping Jacks 35	Half Jumping Jacks 35
60–90 sec. Rest	60–90 sec. Rest	60–90 sec. Rest	60–90 sec. Rest	60–90 sec. Rest
STRETCHES	**STRETCHES**	**LEGS**	**STRETCHES**	**STRETCHES**
Bend Overs	Chest	Walking Lunges 30 yds. (3x)	Chest	Bend Overs
Cross Overs	Lat	High Knees 30 yds. (3x)	Lat	Cross Overs
Inner Thigh	Shoulders	Frog Hops 30 yds. (3x)	Shoulders	Inner Thigh
Forward Lunge	Tricep	Star Hops 15	Tricep	Forward Lunge
Side & Oblique	Partner	Mountain Climbers 15	Partner	Side & Oblique
Hurdler	Arm Rotation	**SPRINTS**	Arm Rotation	Hurdler
Butterfly	60–90 sec. Rest	Intervals (Optional)	60–90 sec. Rest	Butterfly
ITB	**UPPER BODY**	6 Laps = 2400 yds.	**UPPER BODY**	ITB
Thigh	Neck Rotations 20		Neck Rotations 20	Thigh
Calf	Back Contractions 20		Back Contractions 20	Calf
60–90 sec. Rest	Swimmer Exercise 20		Swimmer Exercise 20	60–90 sec. Rest
LEGS	Back Lifts 15		Back Lifts 15	**LEGS**
Lunges 35	60–90 sec. Rest		60–90 sec. Rest	Lunges 35
Squats 45	**PULL-UPS**		**PULL-UPS**	Squats 45
Fire Hydrants 25 (Each Side)	Regular 2-4-6-8-10-8-6-4-2		Regular 2-4-6-8-10-8-6-4-2	Fire Hydrants 25 (Each Side)
Mountain Climber 20	Close Grip 2-4-6-8-6-4-2		Close Grip 2-4-6-8-6-4-2	Mountain Climber 20
The Wall 2:00 min.	Reverse 2-4-6-8-6-4-2		Reverse 2-4-6-8-6-4-2	The Wall 2:00 min.
60–90 sec. Rest	Commandos 2-4-6-4-2		Commandos 2-4-6-4-2	60–90 sec. Rest
CALVES	Behind the Neck 2-4-6-4-2		Behind the Neck 2-4-6-4-2	**CALVES**
Straight (Regular) 75	60–90 sec. Rest		60–90 sec. Rest	Straight (Regular) 75
Toe to Toe 75	**BAR DIPS**		**BAR DIPS**	Toe to Toe 75
Heel to Heel 75	Regular 10		Regular 10	Heel to Heel 75
60–90 sec. Rest	60–90 sec. Rest		60–90 sec. Rest	60–90 sec. Rest
ABDOMINALS	**PUSH-UPS**	**ABDOMINALS**	**PUSH-UPS**	**ABDOMINALS**
Hand to Toes 25	Reg. 2-4-6-8-10-12 ⬇	Clockwork 25-20-15	Reg. 2-4-6-8-10-12 ⬇	Hand to Toes 25
X Sit-Ups 25	Diamond 2-4-6-8-10 ⬇	Hanging Knee Up 25	Diamond 2-4-6-8-10 ⬇	X Sit-Ups 25
Crunches 25	Dive Bombers 2-4-6-8-10 ⬇	Hanging Side Sit-Up 12	Dive Bombers 2-4-6-8-10 ⬇	Crunches 25
Side Sit-Ups 25	8 Count Body Builders 10	Hand to Toe (Short) 25	8 Count Body Builders 10	Side Sit-Ups 25
Obliques 25	Take "After" Supplements	Crunches (Short) 25	Take "After" Supplements	Obliques 25
Flutter Kicks 25	Drink 16 oz. of water	Side Sit-Up (Short) 25	Drink 16 oz. of water	Flutter Kicks 25
Reverse Crunches 25		Obliques (Short) 25		Reverse Crunches 25
Knee Bends 25		Atomic 20		Knee Bends 25
Chest Roll 25		Take "After" Supplements		Chest Roll 25
Take "After" Supplements		Drink 16 oz. of water		Take "After" Supplements
Drink 16 oz. of water				Drink 1 quart of water

MONDAY

MEALS [1][2][3][4] [5]   WATER [1][2][3][4] [5][6][7][8]

SUPPLEMENTS — Before: [3] Electrolyte™ [1] Energy Plus™ — After: [3] Recover™ [2] Restore™

TUESDAY

MEALS [1][2][3][4] [5]   WATER [1][2][3][4] [5][6][7][8]

SUPPLEMENTS — Before: [3] Electrolyte™ [1] Energy Plus™ — After: [3] Recover™ [2] Restore™

WEDNESDAY

MEALS [1][2][3][4] [5]   WATER [1][2][3][4] [5][6][7][8]

SUPPLEMENTS — Before: [3] Electrolyte™ [1] Energy Plus™ — After: [3] Recover™ [2] Restore™

THURSDAY

MEALS [1][2][3][4] [5]   WATER [1][2][3][4] [5][6][7][8]

SUPPLEMENTS — Before: [3] Electrolyte™ [1] Energy Plus™ — After: [3] Recover™ [2] Restore™

FRIDAY

MEALS [1][2][3][4] [5]   WATER [1][2][3][4] [5][6][7][8]

SUPPLEMENTS — Before: [3] Electrolyte™ [1] Energy Plus™ — After: [3] Recover™ [2] Restore™

✓ MONDAY / /

- Take "Before" Supplements
- Drink 16 oz. of water

WARM-UPS
- Jumping Jacks 35
- Running in Place 60 sec.
- Half Jumping Jacks 35
- 60–90 sec. Rest

STRETCHES
- Bend Overs
- Cross Overs
- Inner Thigh
- Forward Lunge
- Side & Oblique
- Hurdler
- Butterfly
- ITB
- Thigh
- Calf
- 60–90 sec. Rest

LEGS
- Lunges 35
- Squats 46
- Fire Hydrants 26 (Each Side)
- Mountain Climber 21
- The Wall 2:00 min.
- 60–90 sec. Rest

CALVES
- Straight (Regular) 75
- Toe to Toe 75
- Heel to Heel 75
- 60–90 sec. Rest

ABDOMINALS
- Hand to Toes 25
- X Sit-Ups 25
- Crunches 25
- Side Sit-Ups 25
- Obliques 25
- Flutter Kicks 25
- Reverse Crunches 25
- Knee Bends 25
- Chest Roll 25
- Take "After" Supplements
- Drink 16 oz. of water

✓ TUESDAY / /

- Take "Before" Supplements
- Drink 16 oz. of water

WARM-UPS
- Jumping Jacks 35
- Running in Place 60 sec.
- Half Jumping Jacks 35
- 60–90 sec. Rest

STRETCHES
- Chest
- Lat
- Shoulders
- Tricep
- Partner
- Arm Rotation
- 60–90 sec. Rest

UPPER BODY
- Neck Rotations 20
- Back Contractions 20
- Swimmer Exercise 20
- Back Lifts 16
- 60–90 sec. Rest

PULL-UPS
- Regular 1-3-5-7-9-11 ⬇
- Close Grip 1-3-5-7-9 ⬇
- Reverse 1-3-5-7-9 ⬇
- Commandos 2-4-6-4-2
- Behind the Neck 2-4-6-4-2
- 60–90 sec. Rest

BAR DIPS
- Regular 11
- 60–90 sec. Rest

PUSH-UPS
- Reg. 2-4-6-8-10-12-14 ⬇
- Diamond 2-4-6-8-10 ⬇
- Dive Bombers 2-4-6-8-10 ⬇
- 8 Count Body Builders 10
- Take "After" Supplements
- Drink 16 oz. of water

✓ WEDNESDAY / /

- Take "Before" Supplements
- Drink 16 oz. of water

WARM-UPS
- Jumping Jacks 35
- Running in Place 60 sec.
- Half Jumping Jacks 35
- 60–90 sec. Rest

LEGS
- Walking Lunges 30 yds. (3x)
- High Knees 30 yds. (3x)
- Frog Hops 30 yds. (3x)
- Star Hops 15
- Mountain Climbers 15

SPRINTS
- Basic Sprints (Optional)
- 3 Sets of Cones
  - First Set — 50%
  - Second Set — 75%
  - Third Set — 100%
- 10 Sets

ABDOMINALS
- Clockwork 25-20-15
- Hanging Knee Up 25
- Hanging Side Sit-Up 12
- Hand to Toe (Short) 25
- Crunches (Short) 25
- Side Sit-Up (Short) 25
- Obliques (Short) 25
- Atomic 22
- Take "After" Supplements
- Drink 16 oz. of water

✓ THURSDAY / /

- Take "Before" Supplements
- Drink 16 oz. of water

WARM-UPS
- Jumping Jacks 35
- Running in Place 60 sec.
- Half Jumping Jacks 35
- 60–90 sec. Rest

STRETCHES
- Chest
- Lat
- Shoulders
- Tricep
- Partner
- Arm Rotation
- 60–90 sec. Rest

UPPER BODY
- Neck Rotations 20
- Back Contractions 20
- Swimmer Exercise 20
- Back Lifts 16
- 60–90 sec. Rest

PULL-UPS
- Regular 1-3-5-7-9-11 ⬇
- Close Grip 1-3-5-7-9 ⬇
- Reverse 1-3-5-7-9 ⬇
- Commandos 2-4-6-4-2
- Behind the Neck 2-4-6-4-2
- 60–90 sec. Rest

BAR DIPS
- Regular 11
- 60–90 sec. Rest

PUSH-UPS
- Reg. 2-4-6-8-10-12-14 ⬇
- Diamond 2-4-6-8-10 ⬇
- Dive Bombers 2-4-6-8-10 ⬇
- 8 Count Body Builders 10
- Take "After" Supplements
- Drink 16 oz. of water

✓ FRIDAY / /

- Take "Before" Supplements
- Drink 16 oz. of water

WARM-UPS
- Jumping Jacks 35
- Running in Place 60 sec.
- Half Jumping Jacks 35
- 60–90 sec. Rest

STRETCHES
- Bend Overs
- Cross Overs
- Inner Thigh
- Forward Lunge
- Side & Oblique
- Hurdler
- Butterfly
- ITB
- Thigh
- Calf
- 60–90 sec. Rest

LEGS
- Lunges 35
- Squats 46
- Fire Hydrants 26 (Each Side)
- Mountain Climber 21
- The Wall 2:00 min.
- 60–90 sec. Rest

CALVES
- Straight (Regular) 75
- Toe to Toe 75
- Heel to Heel 75
- 60–90 sec. Rest

ABDOMINALS
- Hand to Toes 25
- X Sit-Ups 25
- Crunches 25
- Side Sit-Ups 25
- Obliques 25
- Flutter Kicks 25
- Reverse Crunches 25
- Knee Bends 25
- Chest Roll 25
- Take "After" Supplements
- Drink 1 quart of water

MEALS / WATER / SUPPLEMENTS (all days)

MEALS: 1 2 3 4 5
WATER: 1 2 3 4 5 6 7 8

SUPPLEMENTS

Before	After
3 Electrolyte™	3 Recover™
1 Energy Plus™	2 Restore™

WEEK 3   INTERMEDIATE LEVEL

✓ MONDAY / /	✓ TUESDAY / /	✓ WEDNESDAY / /	✓ THURSDAY / /	✓ FRIDAY / /
Take "Before" Supplements	Take "Before" Supplements	Take "Before" Supplements	Take "Before" Supplements	Take "Before" Supplements
Drink 16 oz. of water	Drink 16 oz. of water	Drink 16 oz. of water	Drink 16 oz. of water	Drink 16 oz. of water
WARM-UPS	**WARM-UPS**	**WARM-UPS**	**WARM-UPS**	**WARM-UPS**
Jumping Jacks 35	Jumping Jacks 35	Jumping Jacks 35	Jumping Jacks 35	Jumping Jacks 35
Running in Place 60 sec.	Running in Place 60 sec.	Running in Place 60 sec.	Running in Place 60 sec.	Running in Place 60 sec.
Half Jumping Jacks 35	Half Jumping Jacks 35	Half Jumping Jacks 35	Half Jumping Jacks 35	Half Jumping Jacks 35
60–90 sec. Rest	60–90 sec. Rest	60–90 sec. Rest	60–90 sec. Rest	60–90 sec. Rest
STRETCHES	**STRETCHES**	**LEGS**	**STRETCHES**	**STRETCHES**
Bend Overs	Chest	Walking Lunges 35 yds. (3x)	Chest	Bend Overs
Cross Overs	Lat	High Knees 35 yds. (3x)	Lat	Cross Overs
Inner Thigh	Shoulders	Frog Hops 35 yds. (3x)	Shoulders	Inner Thigh
Forward Lunge	Tricep	Star Hops 15	Tricep	Forward Lunge
Side & Oblique	Partner	Mountain Climbers 15	Partner	Side & Oblique
Hurdler	Arm Rotation	**SPRINTS**	Arm Rotation	Hurdler
Butterfly	60–90 sec. Rest	Intervals (Optional)	*TIMED INTERVALS*	Butterfly
ITB	**UPPER BODY**	6 Laps = 2400 yds.	**UPPER BODY**	ITB
Thigh	Neck Rotations 22		Neck Rotations 60 sec.	Thigh
Calf	Back Contractions 22		Back Contractions 60 sec.	Calf
TIMED INTERVALS	Swimmer Exercise 22		Swimmer Exercise 60 sec.	60–90 sec. Rest
LEGS	Back Lifts 16		Back Lifts 60 sec.	**LEGS**
Lunges 60 sec.	60–90 sec. Rest		60–90 sec. Rest	Lunges 36
Squats 60 sec.	**PULL-UPS**		**PULL-UPS**	Squats 47
Fire Hydrants 60 sec. (Each Side)	Regular 1-3-5-7-9-11 ↓		Regular 60 sec.	Fire Hydrants 27 (Each Side)
Mountain Climber 60 sec.	Close Grip 1-3-5-7-9 ↓		Close Grip 60 sec.	Mountain Climber 22
The Wall 2:15 min.	Reverse 1-3-5-7-9 ↓		Reverse 60 sec.	The Wall 2:15 sec.
60–90 sec. Rest	Commandos 2-4-6-4-2		Commandos 60 sec.	60–90 sec. Rest
CALVES	Behind the Neck 2-4-6-4-2		Behind the Neck 60 sec.	**CALVES**
Straight (Regular) 60 sec.	60–90 sec. Rest		60–90 sec. Rest	Straight (Regular) 75
Toe to Toe 60 sec.	**BAR DIPS**		**BAR DIPS**	Toe to Toe 75
Heel to Heel 60 sec.	Regular 12		Regular 60 sec.	Heel to Heel 75
60–90 sec. Rest	60–90 sec. Rest		60–90 sec. Rest	60–90 sec. Rest
ABDOMINALS	**PUSH-UPS**	**ABDOMINALS**	**PUSH-UPS**	**ABDOMINALS**
Hand to Toes 60 sec.	Reg. 4-6-8-10-12-14-16 ↓	Clockwork 30-25-20	Regular 60 sec.	Hand to Toes 27
X Sit-Ups 60 sec.	Diamond 2-4-6-8-10 ↓	Hanging Knee Up 27	Diamond 60 sec.	X Sit-Ups 27
Crunches 60 sec.	Dive Bombers 2-4-6-8-10 ↓	Hanging Side Sit-Up 13	Dive Bombers 60 sec.	Crunches 27
Side Sit-Ups 60 sec.	8 Count Body Builders 12	Hand to Toe (Short) 27	8 Count Body Builders 60 sec.	Side Sit-Ups 27
Obliques 60 sec.	Take "After" Supplements	Crunches (Short) 27	Take "After" Supplements	Obliques 27
Flutter Kicks 60 sec.	Drink 16 oz. of water	Side Sit-Up (Short) 27	Drink 16 oz. of water	Flutter Kicks 27
Reverse Crunches 60 sec.		Obliques (Short) 27		Reverse Crunches 27
Knee Bends 60 sec.		Atomic 24		Knee Bends 27
Chest Roll 60 sec.		Take "After" Supplements		Chest Roll 27
Take "After" Supplements		Drink 16 oz. of water		Take "After" Supplements
Drink 16 oz. of water				Drink 1 quart of water

WEEK 4 — INTERMEDIATE LEVEL

✓ MONDAY / /	✓ TUESDAY / /	✓ WEDNESDAY / /	✓ THURSDAY / /	✓ FRIDAY / /
Take "Before" Supplements	Take "Before" Supplements	Take "Before" Supplements	Take "Before" Supplements	Take "Before" Supplements
Drink 16 oz. of water	Drink 16 oz. of water	Drink 16 oz. of water	Drink 16 oz. of water	Drink 16 oz. of water
WARM-UPS	**WARM-UPS**	**WARM-UPS**	**WARM-UPS**	**WARM-UPS**
Jumping Jacks 35	Jumping Jacks 35	Jumping Jacks 35	Jumping Jacks 35	Jumping Jacks 35
Running in Place 60 sec.	Running in Place 60 sec.	Running in Place 60 sec.	Running in Place 60 sec.	Running in Place 60 sec.
Half Jumping Jacks 35	Half Jumping Jacks 35	Half Jumping Jacks 35	Half Jumping Jacks 35	Half Jumping Jacks 35
60–90 sec. Rest	60–90 sec. Rest	60–90 sec. Rest	60–90 sec. Rest	60–90 sec. Rest
STRETCHES	**STRETCHES**	**LEGS**	**STRETCHES**	**STRETCHES**
Bend Overs	Chest	Walking Lunges 35 yds. (3x)	Chest	Bend Overs
Cross Overs	Lat	High Knees 35 yds. (3x)	Lat	Cross Overs
Inner Thigh	Shoulders	Frog Hops 35 yds. (3x)	Shoulders	Inner Thigh
Forward Lunge	Tricep	Star Hops 17	Tricep	Forward Lunge
Side & Oblique	Partner	Mountain Climbers 17	Partner	Side & Oblique
Hurdler	Arm Rotation	**SPRINTS**	Arm Rotation	Hurdler
Butterfly	60–90 sec. Rest	Basic Sprints (Optional)	60–90 sec. Rest	Butterfly
ITB	**UPPER BODY**	3 Sets of Cones	**CIRCUIT— UPPER BODY**	ITB
Thigh	Neck Rotations 24	First Set — 50%		Thigh
Calf	Back Contractions 24	Second Set — 75%	**SET 1**	Calf
60–90 sec. Rest	Swimmer Exercise 24	Third Set — 100%	Regular Pull-Ups 10	60–90 sec. Rest
CIRCUIT— LEGS	Back Lifts 16	12 Sets	Bar Dips 10	**LEGS**
	60–90 sec. Rest		Regular Push-Ups 30	Lunges 37
SET 1	**PULL-UPS**		**SET 2**	Squats 48
The Wall 2:15 min.	Regular 1-3-5-7-9-11 ⬇		Close Grip Pull-Ups 10	Fire Hydrants 28 (Each Side)
Frog Hops 30 yds. (4x)	Close Grip 1-3-5-7-9 ⬇		Bar Dips 10	Mountain Climber 23
Hand to Toe 35	Reverse 1-3-5-7-9 ⬇		Diamond Push-Ups 20	The Wall 2:15 min.
SET 2	Commandos 2-4-6-4-2		**SET 3**	60–90 sec. Rest
Walking Lunges 30 yds. (4x)	Behind the Neck 2-4-6-4-2		Reverse Grip Pull-Ups 10	**CALVES**
Star Hops 15	60–90 sec. Rest		Bar Dips 10	Straight (Regular) 80
Side Sit-Ups 35	**BAR DIPS**		Dive Bombers 20	Toe to Toe 80
SET 3	Regular 13		**SET 4**	Heel to Heel 80
Mountain Climbers 15	60–90 sec. Rest		Behind the Neck Pull-Ups 5	60–90 sec. Rest
Regular Calf Raises 75	**PUSH-UPS**		Bar Dips 10	**ABDOMINALS**
Knee Bends 35	Reg. 4-6-8-10-12-14-16-18 ⬇	**ABDOMINALS**	Regular Push-Ups 30	Hand to Toes 30
SET 4	Diamond 1-3-5-7-9-11 ⬇	Clockwork 30-25-20	Take "After" Supplements	X Sit-Ups 30
Fire Hydrants 35 (Each Side)	Dive Bombers 1-3-5-7-9-11 ⬇	Hanging Knee Up 30	Drink 16 oz. of water	Crunches 30
Toe to Toe Calf Raises 75	8 Count Body Builders 12	Hanging Side Sit-Up 15		Side Sit-Ups 30
Crunches 35	Take "After" Supplements	Hand to Toe (Short) 30		Obliques 30
SET 5	Drink 16 oz. of water	Crunches (Short) 30		Flutter Kicks 30
Heel to Heel Calf Raises 75		Side Sit-Up (Short) 30		Reverse Crunches 30
Knee Roll Ups 35		Obliques (Short) 30		Knee Bends 30
Take "After" Supplements		Atomic 26		Chest Roll 30
Drink 16 oz. of water		Take "After" Supplements		Take "After" Supplements
		Drink 16 oz. of water		Drink 1 quart of water

MEALS / WATER

Each day:

MEALS 1 2 3 4 5 **WATER** 1 2 3 4 5 6 7 8

SUPPLEMENTS

Each day:

Before	After
3 Electrolyte™	3 Recover™
1 Energy Plus™	2 Restore™

WEEK 5 — INTERMEDIATE LEVEL

✓ **MONDAY** / /	✓ **TUESDAY** / /	✓ **WEDNESDAY** / /	✓ **THURSDAY** / /	✓ **FRIDAY** / /
Take "Before" Supplements	Take "Before" Supplements	Take "Before" Supplements	Take "Before" Supplements	Take "Before" Supplements
Drink 16 oz. of water	Drink 16 oz. of water	Drink 16 oz. of water	Drink 16 oz. of water	Drink 16 oz. of water
WARM-UPS	**WARM-UPS**	**WARM-UPS**	**WARM-UPS**	**WARM-UPS**
Jumping Jacks 35	Jumping Jacks 35	Jumping Jacks 35	Jumping Jacks 35	Jumping Jacks 35
Running in Place 60 sec.	Running in Place 60 sec.	Running in Place 60 sec.	Running in Place 60 sec.	Running in Place 60 sec.
Half Jumping Jacks 35	Half Jumping Jacks 35	Half Jumping Jacks 35	Half Jumping Jacks 35	Half Jumping Jacks 35
60–90 sec. Rest	60–90 sec. Rest	60–90 sec. Rest	60–90 sec. Rest	60–90 sec. Rest
STRETCHES	**STRETCHES**	**LEGS**	**STRETCHES**	**STRETCHES**
Bend Overs	Chest	Walking Lunges 40 yds. (3x)	Chest	Bend Overs
Cross Overs	Lat	High Knees 40 yds. (3x)	Lat	Cross Overs
Inner Thigh	Shoulders	Frog Hops 40 yds. (3x)	Shoulders	Inner Thigh
Forward Lunge	Tricep	Star Hops 17	Tricep	Forward Lunge
Side & Oblique	Partner	Mountain Climbers 17	Partner	Side & Oblique
Hurdler	Arm Rotation	**SPRINTS**	Arm Rotation	Hurdler
Butterfly	60–90 sec. Rest	Intervals (Optional)	60–90 sec. Rest	Butterfly
ITB	**UPPER BODY**	7 Laps = 2800 yds.	**BURNOUTS— UPPER BODY**	ITB
Thigh	Neck Rotations 26			Thigh
Calf	Back Contractions 26		**SET 1**	Calf
60–90 sec. Rest	Swimmer Exercise 26		Regular Pull-Ups	60–90 sec. Rest
LEGS	Back Lifts 17		Bar Dips	**BURNOUTS— LEGS**
Lunges 38	60–90 sec. Rest		Regular Push-Ups	
Squats 52	**PULL-UPS**		**SET 2**	**SET 1**
Fire Hydrants 32 (Each Side)	Regular 2-4-6-8-10-12 ↓		Close Grip Pull-Ups	The Wall
Mountain Climber 24	Close Grip 2-4-6-8-10 ↓		Bar Dips	Frog Hops
The Wall 2:30 min.	Reverse 2-4-6-8-10 ↓		Diamond Push-Ups	Hand to Toe
60–90 sec. Rest	Commandos 2-4-6-4-2		**SET 3**	**SET 2**
CALVES	Behind the Neck 2-4-6-4-2		Reverse Grip Pull-Ups	Lunges
Straight (Regular) 80	60–90 sec. Rest		Bar Dips	Star Hops
Toe to Toe 80	**BAR DIPS**		Dive Bombers	Side Sit-Ups
Heel to Heel 80	Regular 14		**SET 4**	**SET 3**
60–90 sec. Rest	60–90 sec. Rest		Behind the Neck Pull-Ups	Mountain Climbers
ABDOMINALS	**PUSH-UPS**		Bar Dips	Atomics
Hand to Toes 30	Reg. 6-8-10-12-14-16-18-20 ↓	**ABDOMINALS**	Regular Push-Ups	Knee Bends
X Sit-Ups 30	Diamond 1-3-5-7-9-11 ↓	Clockwork 35-30-25	**SET 5**	**SET 4**
Crunches 30	Dive Bombers 1-3-5-7-9-11 ↓	Hanging Knee Up 30	Commandos	Fire Hydrants (Each Side)
Side Sit-Ups 30	8 Count Body Builders 14	Hanging Side Sit-Up 15	Bar Dips	High Knees
Obliques 30	Take "After" Supplements	Hand to Toe (Short) 30	Diamond Push-Ups	Crunches
Flutter Kicks 30	Drink 16 oz. of water	Crunches (Short) 30	Take "After" Supplements	**SET 5**
Reverse Crunches 30		Side Sit-Up (Short) 30	Drink 16 oz. of water	Calf Raises
Knee Bends 30		Obliques (Short) 30		Sprints
Chest Roll 30		Atomic 28		Knee Roll Ups
Take "After" Supplements		Take "After" Supplements		Take "After" Supplements
Drink 16 oz. of water		Drink 16 oz. of water		Drink 1 quart of water

	MONDAY	TUESDAY	WEDNESDAY	THURSDAY	FRIDAY
MEALS	1 2 3 4 / 5	1 2 3 4 / 5	1 2 3 4 / 5	1 2 3 4 / 5	1 2 3 4 / 5
WATER	1 2 3 4 / 5 6 7 8	1 2 3 4 / 5 6 7 8	1 2 3 4 / 5 6 7 8	1 2 3 4 / 5 6 7 8	1 2 3 4 / 5 6 7 8

SUPPLEMENTS

	Before	After
Monday	3 Electrolyte™ / 1 Energy Plus™	3 Recover™ / 2 Restore™
Tuesday	3 Electrolyte™ / 1 Energy Plus™	3 Recover™ / 2 Restore™
Wednesday	3 Electrolyte™ / 1 Energy Plus™	3 Recover™ / 2 Restore™
Thursday	3 Electrolyte™ / 1 Energy Plus™	3 Recover™ / 2 Restore™
Friday	3 Electrolyte™ / 1 Energy Plus™	3 Recover™ / 2 Restore™

WEEK 6 — INTERMEDIATE LEVEL

✓ MONDAY / /	✓ TUESDAY / /	✓ WEDNESDAY / /	✓ THURSDAY / /	✓ FRIDAY / /
Take "Before" Supplements	Take "Before" Supplements	Take "Before" Supplements	Take "Before" Supplements	Take "Before" Supplements
Drink 16 oz. of water	Drink 16 oz. of water	Drink 16 oz. of water	Drink 16 oz. of water	Drink 16 oz. of water
WARM-UPS	**WARM-UPS**	**WARM-UPS**	**WARM-UPS**	**WARM-UPS**
Jumping Jacks 35	Jumping Jacks 35	Jumping Jacks 35	Jumping Jacks 35	Jumping Jacks 35
Running in Place 60 sec.	Running in Place 60 sec.	Running in Place 60 sec.	Running in Place 60 sec.	Running in Place 60 sec.
Half Jumping Jacks 35	Half Jumping Jacks 35	Half Jumping Jacks 35	Half Jumping Jacks 35	Half Jumping Jacks 35
60–90 sec. Rest	60–90 sec. Rest	60–90 sec. Rest	60–90 sec. Rest	60–90 sec. Rest
STRETCHES	**STRETCHES**	**LEGS**	**STRETCHES**	**STRETCHES**
Bend Overs	Chest	Walking Lunges 30 yds. (4x)	Chest	Bend Overs
Cross Overs	Lat	High Knees 30 yds. (4x)	Lat	Cross Overs
Inner Thigh	Shoulders	Frog Hops 30 yds. (4x)	Shoulders	Inner Thigh
Forward Lunge	Tricep	Star Hops 19	Tricep	Forward Lunge
Side & Oblique	Partner	Mountain Climbers 19	Partner	Side & Oblique
Hurdler	Arm Rotation	**SPRINTS**	Arm Rotation	Hurdler
Butterfly	60–90 sec. Rest	Basic Sprints (Optional)	60–90 sec. Rest	Butterfly
ITB	**UPPER BODY**	3 Sets of Cones	**UPPER BODY**	ITB
Thigh	Neck Rotations 28	First Set — 50%	Neck Rotations 28	Thigh
Calf	Back Contractions 28	Second Set — 75%	Back Contractions 28	Calf
60–90 sec. Rest	Swimmer Exercise 28	Third Set — 100%	Swimmer Exercise 28	60–90 sec. Rest
LEGS	Back Lifts 17	14 Sets	Back Lifts 17	**LEGS**
Lunges 39	60–90 sec. Rest		60–90 sec. Rest	Lunges 39
Squats 53	**PULL-UPS**		**PULL-UPS**	Squats 53
Fire Hydrants 33 (Each Side)	Regular 2-4-6-8-10-12 ⬇		Regular 2-4-6-8-10-12 ⬇	Fire Hydrants 33 (Each Side)
Mountain Climber 25	Close Grip 2-4-6-8-10 ⬇		Close Grip 2-4-6-8-10 ⬇	Mountain Climber 25
The Wall 2:30 min.	Reverse 2-4-6-8-10 ⬇		Reverse 2-4-6-8-10 ⬇	The Wall 2:30 min.
60–90 sec. Rest	Commandos 1-3-5-7-5-3-1		Commandos 1-3-5-7-5-3-1	60–90 sec. Rest
CALVES	Behind the Neck 1-3-5-7-5-3-1		Behind the Neck 1-3-5-7-5-3-1	**CALVES**
Straight (Regular) 85	60–90 sec. Rest		60–90 sec. Rest	Straight (Regular) 85
Toe to Toe 85	**BAR DIPS**		**BAR DIPS**	Toe to Toe 85
Heel to Heel 85	Regular 15		Regular 15	Heel to Heel 85
60–90 sec. Rest	60–90 sec. Rest		60–90 sec. Rest	60–90 sec. Rest
ABDOMINALS	**PUSH-UPS**		**PUSH-UPS**	**ABDOMINALS**
Hand to Toes 35	Reg. 6-8-10-12-14-16-18-20 ⬇	**ABDOMINALS**	Reg. 6-8-10-12-14-16-18-20 ⬇	Hand to Toes 35
X Sit-Ups 35	Diamond 1-3-5-7-9-11 ⬇	Clockwork 35-30-25	Diamond 1-3-5-7-9-11 ⬇	X Sit-Ups 35
Crunches 35	Dive Bombers 1-3-5-7-9-11 ⬇	Hanging Knee Up 35	Dive Bombers 1-3-5-7-9-11 ⬇	Crunches 35
Side Sit-Ups 35	8 Count Body Builders 14	Hanging Side Sit-Up 17	8 Count Body Builders 14	Side Sit-Ups 35
Obliques 35	Take "After" Supplements	Hand to Toe (Short) 35	Take "After" Supplements	Obliques 35
Flutter Kicks 35	Drink 16 oz. of water	Crunches (Short) 35	Drink 16 oz. of water	Flutter Kicks 35
Reverse Crunches 35		Side Sit-Up (Short) 35		Reverse Crunches 35
Knee Bends 35		Obliques (Short) 35		Knee Bends 35
Chest Roll 35		Atomic 30		Chest Roll 35
Take "After" Supplements		Take "After" Supplements		Take "After" Supplements
Drink 16 oz. of water		Drink 16 oz. of water		Drink 1 quart of water

	MONDAY	TUESDAY	WEDNESDAY	THURSDAY	FRIDAY
MEALS	1 2 3 4 5	1 2 3 4 5	1 2 3 4 5	1 2 3 4 5	1 2 3 4 5
WATER	1 2 3 4 5 6 7 8	1 2 3 4 5 6 7 8	1 2 3 4 5 6 7 8	1 2 3 4 5 6 7 8	1 2 3 4 5 6 7 8

SUPPLEMENTS

	Before	After
Monday	3 Electrolyte™ 1 Energy Plus™	3 Recover™ 2 Restore™
Tuesday	3 Electrolyte™ 1 Energy Plus™	3 Recover™ 2 Restore™
Wednesday	3 Electrolyte™ 1 Energy Plus™	3 Recover™ 2 Restore™
Thursday	3 Electrolyte™ 1 Energy Plus™	3 Recover™ 2 Restore™
Friday	3 Electrolyte™ 1 Energy Plus™	3 Recover™ 2 Restore™

✓ MONDAY / /	✓ TUESDAY / /	✓ WEDNESDAY / /	✓ THURSDAY / /	✓ FRIDAY / /
Take "Before" Supplements	Take "Before" Supplements	Take "Before" Supplements	Take "Before" Supplements	Take "Before" Supplements
Drink 16 oz. of water	Drink 16 oz. of water	Drink 16 oz. of water	Drink 16 oz. of water	Drink 16 oz. of water
WARM-UPS	**WARM-UPS**	**WARM-UPS**	**WARM-UPS**	**WARM-UPS**
Jumping Jacks 35	Jumping Jacks 35	Jumping Jacks 35	Jumping Jacks 35	Jumping Jacks 35
Running in Place 60 sec.	Running in Place 60 sec.	Running in Place 60 sec.	Running in Place 60 sec.	Running in Place 60 sec.
Half Jumping Jacks 35	Half Jumping Jacks 35	Half Jumping Jacks 35	Half Jumping Jacks 35	Half Jumping Jacks 35
60–90 sec. Rest	60–90 sec. Rest	60–90 sec. Rest	60–90 sec. Rest	60–90 sec. Rest
STRETCHES	**STRETCHES**	**LEGS**	**STRETCHES**	**STRETCHES**
Bend Overs	Chest	Walking Lunges 35 yds. (4x)	Chest	Bend Overs
Cross Overs	Lat	High Knees 35 yds. (4x)	Lat	Cross Overs
Inner Thigh	Shoulders	Frog Hops 35 yds. (4x)	Shoulders	Inner Thigh
Forward Lunge	Tricep	Star Hops 20	Tricep	Forward Lunge
Side & Oblique	Partner	Mountain Climbers 20	Partner	Side & Oblique
Hurdler	Arm Rotation	**SPRINTS**	Arm Rotation	Hurdler
Butterfly	60–90 sec. Rest	Intervals (Optional)	60–90 sec. Rest	Butterfly
ITB	**UPPER BODY**	7 Laps = 2800 yds.	**UPPER BODY**	ITB
Thigh	Neck Rotations 30		Neck Rotations 30	Thigh
Calf	Back Contractions 30		Back Contractions 30	Calf
60–90 sec. Rest	Swimmer Exercise 30		Swimmer Exercise 30	60–90 sec. Rest
LEGS	Back Lifts 17		Back Lifts 17	**LEGS**
Lunges 40	60–90 sec. Rest		60–90 sec. Rest	Lunges 40
Squats 54	**PULL-UPS**		**PULL-UPS**	Squats 54
Fire Hydrants 34 (Each Side)	Regular 2-4-6-8-10-12 ⬇		Regular 2-4-6-8-10-12 ⬇	Fire Hydrants 34 (Each Side)
Mountain Climber 26	Close Grip 2-4-6-8-10 ⬇		Close Grip 2-4-6-8-10 ⬇	Mountain Climber 26
The Wall 2:30 min.	Reverse 2-4-6-8-10 ⬇		Reverse 2-4-6-8-10 ⬇	The Wall 2:30 min.
60–90 sec. Rest	Commandos 1-3-5-7-5-3-1		Commandos 1-3-5-7-5-3-1	60–90 sec. Rest
CALVES	Behind the Neck 1-3-5-7-5-3-1		Behind the Neck 1-3-5-7-5-3-1	**CALVES**
Straight (Regular) 85	60–90 sec. Rest		60–90 sec. Rest	Straight (Regular) 85
Toe to Toe 85	**BAR DIPS**		**BAR DIPS**	Toe to Toe 85
Heel to Heel 85	Regular 16		Regular 16	Heel to Heel 85
60–90 sec. Rest	60–90 sec. Rest		60–90 sec. Rest	60–90 sec. Rest
ABDOMINALS	**PUSH-UPS**	**ABDOMINALS**	**PUSH-UPS**	**ABDOMINALS**
Hand to Toes 35	Reg. 6-8-10-12-14-16-18-20 ⬇	Clockwork 40-35-30	Reg. 6-8-10-12-14-16-18-20 ⬇	Hand to Toes 35
X Sit-Ups 35	Diamond 1-3-5-7-9-11 ⬇	Hanging Knee Up 35	Diamond 1-3-5-7-9-11 ⬇	X Sit-Ups 35
Crunches 35	Dive Bombers 1-3-5-7-9-11 ⬇	Hanging Side Sit-Up 17	Dive Bombers 1-3-5-7-9-11 ⬇	Crunches 35
Side Sit-Ups 35	8 Count Body Builders 16	Hand to Toe (Short) 35	8 Count Body Builders 16	Side Sit-Ups 35
Obliques 35	Take "After" Supplements	Crunches (Short) 35	Take "After" Supplements	Obliques 35
Flutter Kicks 35	Drink 16 oz. of water	Side Sit-Up (Short) 35	Drink 16 oz. of water	Flutter Kicks 35
Reverse Crunches 35		Obliques (Short) 35		Reverse Crunches 35
Knee Bends 35		Atomic 30		Knee Bends 35
Chest Roll 35		Take "After" Supplements		Chest Roll 35
Take "After" Supplements		Drink 16 oz. of water		Take "After" Supplements
Drink 16 oz. of water				Drink 1 quart of water

MEALS	WATER	MEALS	WATER	MEALS	WATER	MEALS	WATER	MEALS	WATER
1 2 3 4 5	1 2 3 4 5 6 7 8	1 2 3 4 5	1 2 3 4 5 6 7 8	1 2 3 4 5	1 2 3 4 5 6 7 8	1 2 3 4 5	1 2 3 4 5 6 7 8	1 2 3 4 5	1 2 3 4 5 6 7 8

SUPPLEMENTS

Before	After	Before	After	Before	After	Before	After	Before	After
3 Electrolyte™	3 Recover™	3 Electrolyte™	3 Recover™	3 Electrolyte™	3 Recover™	3 Electrolyte™	3 Recover™	3 Electrolyte™	3 Recover™
1 Energy Plus™	2 Restore™	1 Energy Plus™	2 Restore™	1 Energy Plus™	2 Restore™	1 Energy Plus™	2 Restore™	1 Energy Plus™	2 Restore™

✓ MONDAY / /	✓ TUESDAY / /	✓ WEDNESDAY / /	✓ THURSDAY / /	✓ FRIDAY / /
Take "Before" Supplements	Take "Before" Supplements	Take "Before" Supplements	Take "Before" Supplements	Take "Before" Supplements
Drink 16 oz. of water	Drink 16 oz. of water	Drink 16 oz. of water	Drink 16 oz. of water	Drink 16 oz. of water
WARM-UPS	**WARM-UPS**	**WARM-UPS**	**WARM-UPS**	**WARM-UPS**
Jumping Jacks 35	Jumping Jacks 35	Jumping Jacks 35	Jumping Jacks 35	Jumping Jacks 35
Running in Place 60 sec.	Running in Place 60 sec.	Running in Place 60 sec.	Running in Place 60 sec.	Running in Place 60 sec.
Half Jumping Jacks 35	Half Jumping Jacks 35	Half Jumping Jacks 35	Half Jumping Jacks 35	Half Jumping Jacks 35
60–90 sec. Rest	60–90 sec. Rest	60–90 sec. Rest	60–90 sec. Rest	60–90 sec. Rest
STRETCHES	**STRETCHES**	**LEGS**	**STRETCHES**	**STRETCHES**
Bend Overs	Chest	Walking Lunges 40 yds. (4x)	Chest	Bend Overs
Cross Overs	Lat	High Knees 40 yds. (4x)	Lat	Cross Overs
Inner Thigh	Shoulders	Frog Hops 40 yds. (4x)	Shoulders	Inner Thigh
Forward Lunge	Tricep	Star Hops 20	Tricep	Forward Lunge
Side & Oblique	Partner	Mountain Climbers 20	Partner	Side & Oblique
Hurdler	Arm Rotation	**SPRINTS**	Arm Rotation	Hurdler
Butterfly	***TIMED INTERVALS***	Basic Sprints (Optional)	60–90 sec. Rest	Butterfly
ITB	***UPPER BODY***	3 Sets of Cones		ITB
Thigh	Neck Rotations 70 sec.	First Set — 50%	***CIRCUIT—***	Thigh
Calf	Back Contractions 70 sec.	Second Set — 75%	***UPPER BODY***	Calf
TIMED INTERVALS	Swimmer Exercise 70 sec.	Third Set — 100%	**SET 1**	60–90 sec. Rest
LEGS	Back Lifts 70 sec.	16 Sets	Regular Pull-Ups 12	***CIRCUIT—***
Lunges 70 sec.	60–90 sec. Rest		Bar Dips 15	***LEGS***
Squats 70 sec.	**PULL-UPS**		Regular Push-Ups 40	**SET 1**
Fire Hydrants 70 sec. (Each Side)	Regular 70 sec.		**SET 2**	The Wall 2:30 min.
Mountain Climber 70 sec.	Close Grip 70 sec.		Close Grip Pull-Ups 12	Frog Hops 30 yds. (5x)
The Wall 2:45 min.	Reverse 70 sec.		Bar Dips 15	Hand to Toe 40
60–90 sec. Rest	Commandos 70 sec.		Diamond Push-Ups 25	**SET 2**
CALVES	Behind the Neck 70 sec.		**SET 3**	Walking Lunges 30 yds. (5x)
Straight (Regular) 70 sec.	60–90 sec. Rest		Reverse Grip Pull-Ups 12	Star Hops 18
Toe to Toe 70 sec.	**BAR DIPS**		Bar Dips 15	Side Sit-Ups 40
Heel to Heel 70 sec.	Regular 70 sec.		Dive Bombers 25	**SET 3**
60–90 sec. Rest	60–90 sec. Rest		**SET 4**	Mountain Climbers 18
ABDOMINALS	**PUSH-UPS**		Behind the Neck Pull-Ups 7	Regular Calf Raises 85
Hand to Toes 70 sec.	Regular 70 sec.	**ABDOMINALS**	Bar Dips 15	Knee Bends 40
X Sit-Ups 70 sec.	Diamond 70 sec.	Clockwork 40-35-30	Regular Push-Ups 40	**SET 4**
Crunches 70 sec.	Dive Bombers 70 sec.	Hanging Knee Up 40	Take "After" Supplements	Fire Hydrants 40 (Each Side)
Side Sit-Ups 70 sec.	8 Count Body Builders 70 sec.	Hanging Side Sit-Up 20	Drink 16 oz. of water	Toe to Toe Calf Raises 85
Obliques 70 sec.	Take "After" Supplements	Hand to Toe (Short) 40		Crunches 40
Flutter Kicks 70 sec.	Drink 16 oz. of water	Crunches (Short) 40		**SET 5**
Reverse Crunches 70 sec.		Side Sit-Up (Short) 40		Heel to Heel Calf Raises 85
Knee Bends 70 sec.		Obliques (Short) 40		Knee Roll Ups 40
Chest Roll 70 sec.		Atomic 32		Take "After" Supplements
Take "After" Supplements		Take "After" Supplements		Drink 16 oz. of water
Drink 16 oz. of water		Drink 16 oz. of water		

| | **MEALS** | **WATER** | **MEALS** | **WATER** | **MEALS** | **WATER** | **MEALS** | **WATER** | **MEALS** | **WATER** |

MEALS 1 2 3 4 5   WATER 1 2 3 4 5 6 7 8 (each day, Monday–Friday)

SUPPLEMENTS (each day)

Before	After
3 Electrolyte™	**3** Recover™
1 Energy Plus™	**2** Restore™

WEEK 9   INTERMEDIATE LEVEL

✓ MONDAY / /	✓ TUESDAY / /	✓ WEDNESDAY / /	✓ THURSDAY / /	✓ FRIDAY / /
Take "Before" Supplements	Take "Before" Supplements	Take "Before" Supplements	Take "Before" Supplements	Take "Before" Supplements
Drink 16 oz. of water	Drink 16 oz. of water	Drink 16 oz. of water	Drink 16 oz. of water	Drink 16 oz. of water
WARM-UPS	**WARM-UPS**	**WARM-UPS**	**WARM-UPS**	**WARM-UPS**
Jumping Jacks 35	Jumping Jacks 35	Jumping Jacks 35	Jumping Jacks 35	Jumping Jacks 35
Running in Place 60 sec.	Running in Place 60 sec.	Running in Place 60 sec.	Running in Place 60 sec.	Running in Place 60 sec.
Half Jumping Jacks 35	Half Jumping Jacks 35	Half Jumping Jacks 35	Half Jumping Jacks 35	Half Jumping Jacks 35
60–90 sec. Rest	60–90 sec. Rest	60–90 sec. Rest	60–90 sec. Rest	60–90 sec. Rest
STRETCHES	**STRETCHES**	**LEGS**	**STRETCHES**	**STRETCHES**
Bend Overs	Chest	Walking Lunges 40 yds. (4x)	Chest	Bend Overs
Cross Overs	Lat	High Knees 40 yds. (4x)	Lat	Cross Overs
Inner Thigh	Shoulders	Frog Hops 40 yds. (4x)	Shoulders	Inner Thigh
Forward Lunge	Tricep	Star Hops 20	Tricep	Forward Lunge
Side & Oblique	Partner	Mountain Climbers 22	Partner	Side & Oblique
Hurdler	Arm Rotation	**SPRINTS**	Arm Rotation	Hurdler
Butterfly	60–90 sec. Rest	Intervals (Optional)	60–90 sec. Rest	Butterfly
ITB	**UPPER BODY**	7 Laps = 2800 yds.	**UPPER BODY**	ITB
Thigh	Neck Rotations 34		Neck Rotations 34	Thigh
Calf	Back Contractions 34		Back Contractions 34	Calf
60–90 sec. Rest	Swimmer Exercise 34		Swimmer Exercise 34	60–90 sec. Rest
LEGS	Back Lifts 18		Back Lifts 18	**LEGS**
Lunges 42	60–90 sec. Rest		60–90 sec. Rest	Lunges 42
Squats 56	**PULL-UPS**		**PULL-UPS**	Squats 56
Fire Hydrants 36 (Each Side)	Regular 1-3-5-7-9-11-13 ⬇		Regular 1-3-5-7-9-11-13 ⬇	Fire Hydrants 36 (Each Side)
Mountain Climber 28	Close Grip 1-3-5-7-9-11 ⬇		Close Grip 1-3-5-7-9-11 ⬇	Mountain Climber 28
The Wall 2:45 min.	Reverse 1-3-5-7-9-11 ⬇		Reverse 1-3-5-7-9-11 ⬇	The Wall 2:45 min.
60–90 sec. Rest	Commandos 1-3-5-7 ⬇		Commandos 1-3-5-7 ⬇	60–90 sec. Rest
CALVES	Behind the Neck 1-3-5-7 ⬇		Behind the Neck 1-3-5-7 ⬇	**CALVES**
Straight (Regular) 90	60–90 sec. Rest		60–90 sec. Rest	Straight (Regular) 90
Toe to Toe 90	**BAR DIPS**		**BAR DIPS**	Toe to Toe 90
Heel to Heel 90	Regular 18		Regular 18	Heel to Heel 90
60–90 sec. Rest	60–90 sec. Rest		60–90 sec. Rest	60–90 sec. Rest
ABDOMINALS	**PUSH-UPS**		**PUSH-UPS**	**ABDOMINALS**
Hand to Toes 40	Reg. 10-12-14-16-18-20-22 ⬇	**ABDOMINALS**	Reg. 10-12-14-16-18-20-22 ⬇	Hand to Toes 40
X Sit-Ups 40	Diamond 1-3-5-7-9-11 ⬇	Clockwork 45-40-35	Diamond 1-3-5-7-9-11 ⬇	X Sit-Ups 40
Crunches 40	Dive Bombers 1-3-5-7-9-11 ⬇	Hanging Knee Up 40	Dive Bombers 1-3-5-7-9-11 ⬇	Crunches 40
Side Sit-Ups 40	8 Count Body Builders 18	Hanging Side Sit-Up 20	8 Count Body Builders 18	Side Sit-Ups 40
Obliques 40	Take "After" Supplements	Hand to Toe (Short) 40	Take "After" Supplements	Obliques 40
Flutter Kicks 40	Drink 16 oz. of water	Crunches (Short) 40	Drink 16 oz. of water	Flutter Kicks 40
Reverse Crunches 40		Side Sit-Up (Short) 40		Reverse Crunches 40
Knee Bends 40		Obliques (Short) 40		Knee Bends 40
Chest Roll 40		Atomic 34		Chest Roll 40
Take "After" Supplements		Take "After" Supplements		Take "After" Supplements
Drink 16 oz. of water		Drink 16 oz. of water		Drink 1 quart of water

	MONDAY	TUESDAY	WEDNESDAY	THURSDAY	FRIDAY
MEALS	1 2 3 4 5	1 2 3 4 5	1 2 3 4 5	1 2 3 4 5	1 2 3 4 5
WATER	1 2 3 4 5 6 7 8	1 2 3 4 5 6 7 8	1 2 3 4 5 6 7 8	1 2 3 4 5 6 7 8	1 2 3 4 5 6 7 8

SUPPLEMENTS (each day)

	Before	After
	3 Electrolyte™	**3** Recover™
	1 Energy Plus™	**2** Restore™

✓ MONDAY / /	✓ TUESDAY / /	✓ WEDNESDAY / /	✓ THURSDAY / /	✓ FRIDAY / /
Take "Before" Supplements	Take "Before" Supplements	Take "Before" Supplements	Take "Before" Supplements	Take "Before" Supplements
Drink 16 oz. of water	Drink 16 oz. of water	Drink 16 oz. of water	Drink 16 oz. of water	Drink 16 oz. of water
WARM-UPS	**WARM-UPS**	**WARM-UPS**	**WARM-UPS**	**WARM-UPS**
Jumping Jacks 35	Jumping Jacks 35	Jumping Jacks 35	Jumping Jacks 35	Jumping Jacks 35
Running in Place 60 sec.	Running in Place 60 sec.	Running in Place 60 sec.	Running in Place 60 sec.	Running in Place 60 sec.
Half Jumping Jacks 35	Half Jumping Jacks 35	Half Jumping Jacks 35	Half Jumping Jacks 35	Half Jumping Jacks 35
60–90 sec. Rest	60–90 sec. Rest	60–90 sec. Rest	60–90 sec. Rest	60–90 sec. Rest
STRETCHES	**STRETCHES**	**LEGS**	**STRETCHES**	**STRETCHES**
Bend Overs	Chest	Walking Lunges 40 yds. (4x)	Chest	Bend Overs
Cross Overs	Lat	High Knees 40 yds. (4x)	Lat	Cross Overs
Inner Thigh	Shoulders	Frog Hops 40 yds. (4x)	Shoulders	Inner Thigh
Forward Lunge	Tricep	Star Hops 20	Tricep	Forward Lunge
Side & Oblique	Partner	Mountain Climbers 22	Partner	Side & Oblique
Hurdler	Arm Rotation	**SPRINTS**	Arm Rotation	Hurdler
Butterfly	60–90 sec. Rest	Basic Sprints (Optional)	60–90 sec. Rest	Butterfly
ITB	**UPPER BODY**	3 Sets of Cones	**BURNOUTS— UPPER BODY**	ITB
Thigh	Neck Rotations 36	First Set — 50%		Thigh
Calf	Back Contractions 36	Second Set — 75%	**SET 1**	Calf
60–90 sec. Rest	Swimmer Exercise 36	Third Set — 100%	Regular Pull-Ups	60–90 sec. Rest
BURNOUTS— LEGS	Back Lifts 18	18 Sets	Bar Dips	**LEGS**
	60–90 sec. Rest		Regular Push-Ups	Lunges 43
SET 1	**PULL-UPS**		**SET 2**	Squats 57
The Wall	Regular 1-3-5-7-9-11-13 ⬇		Close Grip Pull-Ups	Fire Hydrants 37 (Each Side)
Frog Hops	Close Grip 1-3-5-7-9-11 ⬇		Bar Dips	Mountain Climber 29
Hand to Toe	Reverse 1-3-5-7-9-11 ⬇		Diamond Push-Ups	The Wall 2:45 min.
SET 2	Commandos 1-3-5-7 ⬇		**SET 3**	60–90 sec. Rest
Lunges	Behind the Neck 1-3-5-7 ⬇		Reverse Grip Pull-Ups	**CALVES**
Star Hops	60–90 sec. Rest		Bar Dips	Straight (Regular) 95
Side Sit-Ups	**BAR DIPS**		Dive Bombers	Toe to Toe 95
SET 3	Regular 19		**SET 4**	Heel to Heel 95
Mountain Climbers	60–90 sec. Rest		Behind the Neck Pull-Ups	60–90 sec. Rest
Atomics	**PUSH-UPS**		Bar Dips	**ABDOMINALS**
Knee Bends	Reg. 10-12-14-16-18-20-22 ⬇	**ABDOMINALS**	Regular Push-Ups	Hand to Toes 45
SET 4	Diamond 2-4-6-8-10-12 ⬇	Clockwork 45-40-35	**SET 5**	X Sit-Ups 45
Fire Hydrants (Each Side)	Dive Bombers 4-6-8-10-12 ⬇	Hanging Knee Up 45	Commandos	Crunches 45
High Knees	8 Count Body Builders 18	Hanging Side Sit-Up 22	Bar Dips	Side Sit-Ups 45
Crunches	Take "After" Supplements	Hand to Toe (Short) 45	Diamond Push-Ups	Obliques 45
SET 5	Drink 16 oz. of water	Crunches (Short) 45	Take "After" Supplements	Flutter Kicks 45
Calf Raises		Side Sit-Up (Short) 45	Drink 16 oz. of water	Reverse Crunches 45
Sprints		Obliques (Short) 45		Knee Bends 45
Knee Roll Ups		Atomic 36		Chest Roll 45
Take "After" Supplements		Take "After" Supplements		Take "After" Supplements
Drink 1 quart of water		Drink 16 oz. of water		Drink 1 quart of water

MEALS 1 2 3 4 5 **WATER** 1 2 3 4 5 6 7 8
SUPPLEMENTS — Before: 3 Electrolyte™ 1 Energy Plus™ / After: 3 Recover™ 2 Restore™

MEALS 1 2 3 4 5 **WATER** 1 2 3 4 5 6 7 8
SUPPLEMENTS — Before: 3 Electrolyte™ 1 Energy Plus™ / After: 3 Recover™ 2 Restore™

MEALS 1 2 3 4 5 **WATER** 1 2 3 4 5 6 7 8
SUPPLEMENTS — Before: 3 Electrolyte™ 1 Energy Plus™ / After: 3 Recover™ 2 Restore™

MEALS 1 2 3 4 5 **WATER** 1 2 3 4 5 6 7 8
SUPPLEMENTS — Before: 3 Electrolyte™ 1 Energy Plus™ / After: 3 Recover™ 2 Restore™

MEALS 1 2 3 4 5 **WATER** 1 2 3 4 5 6 7 8
SUPPLEMENTS — Before: 3 Electrolyte™ 1 Energy Plus™ / After: 3 Recover™ 2 Restore™

WEEK 11 — INTERMEDIATE LEVEL

✓ MONDAY / /	✓ TUESDAY / /	✓ WEDNESDAY / /	✓ THURSDAY / /	✓ FRIDAY / /
Take "Before" Supplements	Take "Before" Supplements	Take "Before" Supplements	Take "Before" Supplements	Take "Before" Supplements
Drink 16 oz. of water	Drink 16 oz. of water	Drink 16 oz. of water	Drink 16 oz. of water	Drink 16 oz. of water
WARM-UPS	**WARM-UPS**	**WARM-UPS**	**WARM-UPS**	**WARM-UPS**
Jumping Jacks 35	Jumping Jacks 35	Jumping Jacks 35	Jumping Jacks 35	Jumping Jacks 35
Running in Place 60 sec.	Running in Place 60 sec.	Running in Place 60 sec.	Running in Place 60 sec.	Running in Place 60 sec.
Half Jumping Jacks 35	Half Jumping Jacks 35	Half Jumping Jacks 35	Half Jumping Jacks 35	Half Jumping Jacks 35
60–90 sec. Rest	60–90 sec. Rest	60–90 sec. Rest	60–90 sec. Rest	60–90 sec. Rest
STRETCHES	**STRETCHES**	**LEGS**	**STRETCHES**	**STRETCHES**
Bend Overs	Chest	Walking Lunges 40 yds. (4x)	Chest	Bend Overs
Cross Overs	Lat	High Knees 40 yds. (4x)	Lat	Cross Overs
Inner Thigh	Shoulders	Frog Hops 40 yds. (4x)	Shoulders	Inner Thigh
Forward Lunge	Tricep	Star Hops 20	Tricep	Forward Lunge
Side & Oblique	Partner	Mountain Climbers 25	Partner	Side & Oblique
Hurdler	Arm Rotation	**SPRINTS**	Arm Rotation	Hurdler
Butterfly	60–90 sec. Rest	Intervals (Optional)	60–90 sec. Rest	Butterfly
ITB	**UPPER BODY**	8 Laps = 3200 yds.	**UPPER BODY**	ITB
Thigh	Neck Rotations 38		Neck Rotations 38	Thigh
Calf	Back Contractions 38		Back Contractions 38	Calf
60–90 sec. Rest	Swimmer Exercise 38		Swimmer Exercise 38	60–90 sec. Rest
LEGS	Back Lifts 18		Back Lifts 18	**LEGS**
Lunges 44	60–90 sec. Rest		60–90 sec. Rest	Lunges 44
Squats 58	**PULL-UPS**		**PULL-UPS**	Squats 58
Fire Hydrants 38 (Each Side)	Regular 1-3-5-7-9-11-13 ⬇		Regular 1-3-5-7-9-11-13 ⬇	Fire Hydrants 38 (Each Side)
Mountain Climber 30	Close Grip 1-3-5-7-9-11 ⬇		Close Grip 1-3-5-7-9-11 ⬇	Mountain Climber 30
The Wall 3:00 min.	Reverse 1-3-5-7-9-11 ⬇		Reverse 1-3-5-7-9-11 ⬇	The Wall 3:00 min.
60–90 sec. Rest	Commandos 1-3-5-7 ⬇		Commandos 1-3-5-7 ⬇	60–90 sec. Rest
CALVES	Behind the Neck v1-3-5-7 ⬇		Behind the Neck 1-3-5-7 ⬇	**CALVES**
Straight (Regular) 95	60–90 sec. Rest		60–90 sec. Rest	Straight (Regular) 95
Toe to Toe 95	**BAR DIPS**		**BAR DIPS**	Toe to Toe 95
Heel to Heel 95	Regular 20		Regular 20	Heel to Heel 95
60–90 sec. Rest	60–90 sec. Rest		60–90 sec. Rest	60–90 sec. Rest
ABDOMINALS	**PUSH-UPS**		**PUSH-UPS**	**ABDOMINALS**
Hand to Toes 45	Reg. 12-14-16-18-20-22-24 ⬇	**ABDOMINALS**	Reg. 12-14-16-18-20-22-24 ⬇	Hand to Toes 45
X Sit-Ups 45	Diamond 4-6-8-10-12 ⬇	Clockwork 50-45-40	Diamond 4-6-8-10-12 ⬇	X Sit-Ups 45
Crunches 45	Dive Bombers 4-6-8-10-12 ⬇	Hanging Knee Up 45	Dive Bombers 4-6-8-10-12 ⬇	Crunches 45
Side Sit-Ups 45	8 Count Body Builders 20	Hanging Side Sit-Up 22	8 Count Body Builders 20	Side Sit-Ups 45
Obliques 45	Take "After" Supplements	Hand to Toe (Short) 45	Take "After" Supplements	Obliques 45
Flutter Kicks 45	Drink 16 oz. of water	Crunches (Short) 45	Drink 16 oz. of water	Flutter Kicks 45
Reverse Crunches 45		Side Sit-Up (Short) 45		Reverse Crunches 45
Knee Bends 45		Obliques (Short) 45		Knee Bends 45
Chest Roll 45		Atomic 38		Chest Roll 45
Take "After" Supplements		Take "After" Supplements		Take "After" Supplements
Drink 16 oz. of water		Drink 16 oz. of water		Drink 1 quart of water

MONDAY
- **MEALS:** 1 2 3 4 5
- **WATER:** 1 2 3 4 5 6 7 8
- **SUPPLEMENTS**
  - Before: 3 Electrolyte™ | 1 Energy Plus™
  - After: 3 Recover™ | 2 Restore™

TUESDAY
- **MEALS:** 1 2 3 4 5
- **WATER:** 1 2 3 4 5 6 7 8
- **SUPPLEMENTS**
  - Before: 3 Electrolyte™ | 1 Energy Plus™
  - After: 3 Recover™ | 2 Restore™

WEDNESDAY
- **MEALS:** 1 2 3 4 5
- **WATER:** 1 2 3 4 5 6 7 8
- **SUPPLEMENTS**
  - Before: 3 Electrolyte™ | 1 Energy Plus™
  - After: 3 Recover™ | 2 Restore™

THURSDAY
- **MEALS:** 1 2 3 4 5
- **WATER:** 1 2 3 4 5 6 7 8
- **SUPPLEMENTS**
  - Before: 3 Electrolyte™ | 1 Energy Plus™
  - After: 3 Recover™ | 2 Restore™

FRIDAY
- **MEALS:** 1 2 3 4 5
- **WATER:** 1 2 3 4 5 6 7 8
- **SUPPLEMENTS**
  - Before: 3 Electrolyte™ | 1 Energy Plus™
  - After: 3 Recover™ | 2 Restore™

WEEK 12 — INTERMEDIATE LEVEL

✓ MONDAY / /	✓ TUESDAY / /	✓ WEDNESDAY / /	✓ THURSDAY / /	✓ FRIDAY / /
Take "Before" Supplements	Take "Before" Supplements	Take "Before" Supplements	Take "Before" Supplements	Take "Before" Supplements
Drink 16 oz. of water	Drink 16 oz. of water	Drink 16 oz. of water	Drink 16 oz. of water	Drink 16 oz. of water
WARM-UPS	**WARM-UPS**	**WARM-UPS**	**WARM-UPS**	**WARM-UPS**
Jumping Jacks 35	Jumping Jacks 35	Jumping Jacks 35	Jumping Jacks 35	Jumping Jacks 35
Running in Place 60 sec.	Running in Place 60 sec.	Running in Place 60 sec.	Running in Place 60 sec.	Running in Place 60 sec.
Half Jumping Jacks 35	Half Jumping Jacks 35	Half Jumping Jacks 35	Half Jumping Jacks 35	Half Jumping Jacks 35
60–90 sec. Rest	60–90 sec. Rest	60–90 sec. Rest	60–90 sec. Rest	60–90 sec. Rest
STRETCHES	**STRETCHES**	**LEGS**	**STRETCHES**	**STRETCHES**
Bend Overs	Chest	Walking Lunges 40 yds. (4x)	Chest	Bend Overs
Cross Overs	Lat	High Knees 40 yds. (4x)	Lat	Cross Overs
Inner Thigh	Shoulders	Frog Hops 40 yds. (4x)	Shoulders	Inner Thigh
Forward Lunge	Tricep	Star Hops 20	Tricep	Forward Lunge
Side & Oblique	Partner	Mountain Climbers 25	Partner	Side & Oblique
Hurdler	Arm Rotation	**SPRINTS**	Arm Rotation	Hurdler
Butterfly	60–90 sec. Rest	Basic Sprints (Optional)	60–90 sec. Rest	Butterfly
ITB	**UPPER BODY**	3 Sets of Cones	**UPPER BODY**	ITB
Thigh	Neck Rotations 40	First Set — 50%	Neck Rotations 40	Thigh
Calf	Back Contractions 40	Second Set — 75%	Back Contractions 40	Calf
60–90 sec. Rest	Swimmer Exercise 40	Third Set — 100%	Swimmer Exercise 40	60–90 sec. Rest
LEGS	Back Lifts 20	20 Sets	Back Lifts 20	**LEGS**
Lunges 45	60–90 sec. Rest		60–90 sec. Rest	Lunges 45
Squats 60	**PULL-UPS**		**PULL-UPS**	Squats 60
Fire Hydrants 40 (Each Side)	Regular 2-4-6-8-10-12-14 ↓		Regular 2-4-6-8-10-12-14 ↓	Fire Hydrants 40 (Each Side)
Mountain Climber 30	Close Grip 2-4-6-8-10-12 ↓		Close Grip 2-4-6-8-10-12 ↓	Mountain Climber 30
The Wall 3:00 min.	Reverse 2-4-6-8-10-12 ↓		Reverse 2-4-6-8-10-12 ↓	The Wall 3:00 min.
60–90 sec. Rest	Commandos 2-4-6-8-6-4-2		Commandos 2-4-6-8-6-4-2	60–90 sec. Rest
CALVES	Behind the Neck 2-4-6-8-6-4-2		Behind the Neck 2-4-6-8-6-4-2	**CALVES**
Straight (Regular) 100	60–90 sec. Rest		60–90 sec. Rest	Straight (Regular) 100
Toe to Toe 100	**BAR DIPS**		**BAR DIPS**	Toe to Toe 100
Heel to Heel 100	Regular 20		Regular 20	Heel to Heel 100
60–90 sec. Rest	60–90 sec. Rest		60–90 sec. Rest	60–90 sec. Rest
ABDOMINALS	**PUSH-UPS**		**PUSH-UPS**	**ABDOMINALS**
Hand to Toes 50	Reg. 12-14-16-18-20-22-24 ↓	**ABDOMINALS**	Reg. 12-14-16-18-20-22-24 ↓	Hand to Toes 50
X Sit-Ups 50	Diamond 2-4-6-8-10-12 ↓	Clockwork 50-45-40	Diamond 2-4-6-8-10-12 ↓	X Sit-Ups 50
Crunches 50	Dive Bombers 4-6-8-10-12 ↓	Hanging Knee Up 50	Dive Bombers 4-6-8-10-12 ↓	Crunches 50
Side Sit-Ups 50	8 Count Body Builders 20	Hanging Side Sit-Up 25	8 Count Body Builders 20	Side Sit-Ups 50
Obliques 50	Take "After" Supplements	Hand to Toe (Short) 50	Take "After" Supplements	Obliques 50
Flutter Kicks 50	Drink 16 oz. of water	Crunches (Short) 50	Drink 16 oz. of water	Flutter Kicks 50
Reverse Crunches 50		Side Sit-Up (Short) 50		Reverse Crunches 50
Knee Bends 50		Obliques (Short) 50		Knee Bends 50
Chest Roll 50		Atomic 40		Chest Roll 50
Take "After" Supplements		Take "After" Supplements		Take "After" Supplements
Drink 16 oz. of water		Drink 16 oz. of water		Drink 1 quart of water

	MEALS	WATER		MEALS	WATER		MEALS	WATER		MEALS	WATER		MEALS	WATER
	1 2 3 4 5	1 2 3 4 5 6 7 8		1 2 3 4 5	1 2 3 4 5 6 7 8		1 2 3 4 5	1 2 3 4 5 6 7 8		1 2 3 4 5	1 2 3 4 5 6 7 8		1 2 3 4 5	1 2 3 4 5 6 7 8

SUPPLEMENTS

Before	After	Before	After	Before	After	Before	After	Before	After
3 Electrolyte™	**3** Recover™	**3** Electrolyte™	**3** Recover™	**3** Electrolyte™	**3** Recover™	**3** Electrolyte™	**3** Recover™	**3** Electrolyte™	**3** Recover™
1 Energy Plus™	**2** Restore™	**1** Energy Plus™	**2** Restore™	**1** Energy Plus™	**2** Restore™	**1** Energy Plus™	**2** Restore™	**1** Energy Plus™	**2** Restore™

✓ **MONDAY** / /	✓ **TUESDAY** / /	✓ **WEDNESDAY** / /	✓ **THURSDAY** / /	✓ **FRIDAY** / /
Take "Before" Supplements	Take "Before" Supplements	Take "Before" Supplements	Take "Before" Supplements	Take "Before" Supplements
Drink 16 oz. of water	Drink 16 oz. of water	Drink 16 oz. of water	Drink 16 oz. of water	Drink 16 oz. of water
WARM-UPS	**WARM-UPS**	**WARM-UPS**	**WARM-UPS**	**WARM-UPS**
Jumping Jacks 40	Jumping Jacks 40	Jumping Jacks 40	Jumping Jacks 40	Jumping Jacks 40
Running in Place 60 sec.	Running in Place 60 sec.	Running in Place 60 sec.	Running in Place 60 sec.	Running in Place 60 sec.
Half Jumping Jacks 40	Half Jumping Jacks 40	Half Jumping Jacks 40	Half Jumping Jacks 40	Half Jumping Jacks 40
60–90 sec. Rest	60–90 sec. Rest	60–90 sec. Rest	60–90 sec. Rest	60–90 sec. Rest
STRETCHES	**STRETCHES**	**LEGS**	**STRETCHES**	**STRETCHES**
Bend Overs	Chest	Walking Lunges 40 yds. (4x)	Chest	Bend Overs
Cross Overs	Lat	High Knees 40 yds. (4x)	Lat	Cross Overs
Inner Thigh	Shoulders	Frog Hops 40 yds. (4x)	Shoulders	Inner Thigh
Forward Lunge	Tricep	Star Hops 20	Tricep	Forward Lunge
Side & Oblique	Partner	Mountain Climbers 25	Partner	Side & Oblique
Hurdler	Arm Rotation	**SPRINTS**	Arm Rotation	Hurdler
Butterfly	60–90 sec. Rest	Basic Sprints (Optional)	60–90 sec. Rest	Butterfly
ITB	**UPPER BODY**	3 Sets of Cones	***BURNOUTS— UPPER BODY***	ITB
Thigh	Neck Rotations 40	First Set — 50%		Thigh
Calf	Back Contractions 40	Second Set — 75%	**SET 1**	Calf
60–90 sec. Rest	Swimmer Exercise 40	Third Set — 100%	Regular Pull-Ups	60–90 sec. Rest
LEGS	Back Lifts 20	20 Sets	Bar Dips	***BURNOUTS— LEGS***
Lunges 45	60–90 sec. Rest		Regular Push-Ups	
Squats 60	**PULL-UPS**		**SET 2**	**SET 1**
Fire Hydrants 40 (Each Side)	Regular 2-4-6-8-10-12-14 ⬇		Close Grip Pull-Ups	The Wall
Mountain Climber 30	Close Grip 2-4-6-8-10-12 ⬇		Bar Dips	Frog Hops
The Wall 3:00 min.	Reverse 2-4-6-8-10-12 ⬇		Diamond Push-Ups	Hand to Toe
60–90 sec. Rest	Commandos 2-4-6-8-6-4-2		**SET 3**	**SET 2**
CALVES	Behind the Neck 2-4-6-8-6-4-2		Reverse Grip Pull-Ups	Lunges
Straight (Regular) 100	60–90 sec. Rest		Bar Dips	Star Hops
Toe to Toe 100	**BAR DIPS**		Dive Bombers	Side Sit-Ups
Heel to Heel 100	Regular 20		**SET 4**	**SET 3**
60–90 sec. Rest	60–90 sec. Rest		Behind the Neck Pull-Ups	Mountain Climbers
ABDOMINALS	**PUSH-UPS**		Bar Dips	Atomics
Hand to Toes 50	Reg. 12-14-16-18-20-22-24 ⬇	**ABDOMINALS**	Regular Push-Ups	Knee Bends
X Sit-Ups 50	Diamond 2-4-6-8-10-12 ⬇	Clockwork 50-45-40	**SET 5**	**SET 4**
Crunches 50	Dive Bombers 4-6-8-10-12 ⬇	Hanging Knee Up 50	Commandos	Fire Hydrants (Each Side)
Side Sit-Ups 50	8 Count Body Builders 20	Hanging Side Sit-Up 25	Bar Dips	High Knees
Obliques 50	Take "After" Supplements	Hand to Toe (Short) 50	Diamond Push-Ups	Crunches
Flutter Kicks 50	Drink 16 oz. of water	Crunches (Short) 50	Take "After" Supplements	**SET 5**
Reverse Crunches 50		Side Sit-Up (Short) 50	Drink 16 oz. of water	Calf Raises
Knee Bends 50		Obliques (Short) 50		Sprints
Chest Roll 50		Atomic 40		Knee Roll Ups
Take "After" Supplements		Take "After" Supplements		Take "After" Supplements
Drink 16 oz. of water		Drink 16 oz. of water		Drink 1 quart of water

MEALS **WATER**	**MEALS** **WATER**	**MEALS** **WATER**	**MEALS** **WATER**	**MEALS** **WATER**
1 2 3 4 1 2 3 4 5 5 6 7 8	1 2 3 4 1 2 3 4 5 5 6 7 8	1 2 3 4 1 2 3 4 5 5 6 7 8	1 2 3 4 1 2 3 4 5 5 6 7 8	1 2 3 4 1 2 3 4 5 5 6 7 8
SUPPLEMENTS	**SUPPLEMENTS**	**SUPPLEMENTS**	**SUPPLEMENTS**	**SUPPLEMENTS**
Before: 3 Electrolyte™, 1 Energy Plus™ After: 3 Recover™, 2 Restore™	Before: 3 Electrolyte™, 1 Energy Plus™ After: 3 Recover™, 2 Restore™	Before: 3 Electrolyte™, 1 Energy Plus™ After: 3 Recover™, 2 Restore™	Before: 3 Electrolyte™, 1 Energy Plus™ After: 3 Recover™, 2 Restore™	Before: 3 Electrolyte™, 1 Energy Plus™ After: 3 Recover™, 2 Restore™

WEEK 2 — ADVANCED LEVEL

✓ MONDAY / /	✓ TUESDAY / /	✓ WEDNESDAY / /	✓ THURSDAY / /	✓ FRIDAY / /
Take "Before" Supplements	Take "Before" Supplements	Take "Before" Supplements	Take "Before" Supplements	Take "Before" Supplements
Drink 16 oz. of water	Drink 16 oz. of water	Drink 16 oz. of water	Drink 16 oz. of water	Drink 16 oz. of water
WARM-UPS	**WARM-UPS**	**WARM-UPS**	**WARM-UPS**	**WARM-UPS**
Jumping Jacks 45	Jumping Jacks 45	Jumping Jacks 45	Jumping Jacks 45	Jumping Jacks 45
Running in Place 60 sec.	Running in Place 60 sec.	Running in Place 60 sec.	Running in Place 60 sec.	Running in Place 60 sec.
Half Jumping Jacks 45	Half Jumping Jacks 45	Half Jumping Jacks 45	Half Jumping Jacks 45	Half Jumping Jacks 45
60–90 sec. Rest	60–90 sec. Rest	60–90 sec. Rest	60–90 sec. Rest	60–90 sec. Rest
STRETCHES	**STRETCHES**	**LEGS**	**STRETCHES**	**STRETCHES**
Bend Overs	Chest	Walking Lunges 40 yds. (4x)	Chest	Bend Overs
Cross Overs	Lat	High Knees 40 yds. (4x)	Lat	Cross Overs
Inner Thigh	Shoulders	Frog Hops 40 yds. (4x)	Shoulders	Inner Thigh
Forward Lunge	Tricep	Star Hops 20	Tricep	Forward Lunge
Side & Oblique	Partner	Mountain Climbers 25	Partner	Side & Oblique
Hurdler	Arm Rotation	**SPRINTS**	Arm Rotation	Hurdler
Butterfly	60–90 sec. Rest	Intervals (Optional)	60–90 sec. Rest	Butterfly
ITB	***CIRCUIT— UPPER BODY***	8 Laps = 3200 yds.	**UPPER BODY**	ITB
Thigh	**SET 1**		Neck Rotations 40	Thigh
Calf	Regular Pull-Ups 20		Back Contractions 40	Calf
60–90 sec. Rest	Bar Dips 30		Swimmer Exercise 40	60–90 sec. Rest
LEGS	Regular Push-Ups 55		Back Lifts 20	***CIRCUIT— LEGS***
Lunges 45	**SET 2**		60–90 sec. Rest	**SET 1**
Squats 60	Close Grip Pull-Ups 20		**PULL-UPS**	The Wall 3:00 min.
Fire Hydrants 40 (Each Side)	Bar Dips 30		Regular 2-4-6-8-10-12-14 ⬇	Frog Hops 40 yds. (5x)
Mountain Climber 30	Diamond Push-Ups 40		Close Grip 2-4-6-8-10-12 ⬇	Hand to Toe 40
The Wall 3:00 min.	**SET 3**		Reverse 2-4-6-8-10-12 ⬇	**SET 2**
60–90 sec. Rest	Reverse Grip Pull-Ups 20		Commandos 2-4-6-8-6-4-2	Walking Lunges 40 yds. (5x)
CALVES	Bar Dips 30		Behind the Neck 2-4-6-8-6-4-2	Star Hops 20
Straight (Regular) 100	Dive Bombers 40		60–90 sec. Rest	Side Sit-Ups 45
Toe to Toe 100	**SET 4**		**BAR DIPS**	**SET 3**
Heel to Heel 100	Behind the Neck Pull-Ups 15		Regular 20	Mountain Climbers 20
60–90 sec. Rest	Bar Dips 30		60–90 sec. Rest	Regular Calf Raises 95
ABDOMINALS	Regular Push-Ups 55	**ABDOMINALS**	**PUSH-UPS**	Knee Bends 45
Hand to Toes 50	Take "After" Supplements	Clockwork 50-45-40	Reg. 12-14-16-18-20-22-24 ⬇	**SET 4**
X Sit-Ups 50	Drink 16 oz. of water	Hanging Knee Up 50	Diamond 2-4-6-8-10-12 ⬇	Fire Hydrants 45 (Each Side)
Crunches 50		Hanging Side Sit-Up 25	Dive Bombers 2-4-6-8-10-12 ⬇	Toe to Toe Calf Raises 95
Side Sit-Ups 50		Hand to Toe (Short) 50	8 Count Body Builders 20	Crunches 45
Obliques 50		Crunches (Short) 50	Take "After" Supplements	**SET 5**
Flutter Kicks 50		Side Sit-Up (Short) 50	Drink 16 oz. of water	Heel to Heel Calf Raises 95
Reverse Crunches 50		Obliques (Short) 50		Knee Roll Ups 45
Knee Bends 50		Atomic 40		Take "After" Supplements
Chest Roll 50		Take "After" Supplements		Drink 16 oz. of water
Take "After" Supplements		Drink 16 oz. of water		
Drink 16 oz. of water				

MEALS / WATER

	MONDAY	TUESDAY	WEDNESDAY	THURSDAY	FRIDAY
MEALS	1 2 3 4 / 5	1 2 3 4 / 5	1 2 3 4 / 5	1 2 3 4 / 5	1 2 3 4 / 5
WATER	1 2 3 4 / 5 6 7 8	1 2 3 4 / 5 6 7 8	1 2 3 4 / 5 6 7 8	1 2 3 4 / 5 6 7 8	1 2 3 4 / 5 6 7 8

SUPPLEMENTS

	Before	After
Monday	3 Electrolyte™ / 1 Energy Plus™	3 Recover™ / 2 Restore™
Tuesday	3 Electrolyte™ / 1 Energy Plus™	3 Recover™ / 2 Restore™
Wednesday	3 Electrolyte™ / 1 Energy Plus™	3 Recover™ / 2 Restore™
Thursday	3 Electrolyte™ / 1 Energy Plus™	3 Recover™ / 2 Restore™
Friday	3 Electrolyte™ / 1 Energy Plus™	3 Recover™ / 2 Restore™

WEEK 3 — ADVANCED LEVEL

✓ MONDAY / /	✓ TUESDAY / /	✓ WEDNESDAY / /	✓ THURSDAY / /	✓ FRIDAY / /
Take "Before" Supplements	Take "Before" Supplements	Take "Before" Supplements	Take "Before" Supplements	Take "Before" Supplements
Drink 16 oz. of water	Drink 16 oz. of water	Drink 16 oz. of water	Drink 16 oz. of water	Drink 16 oz. of water
WARM-UPS	**WARM-UPS**	**WARM-UPS**	**WARM-UPS**	**WARM-UPS**
Jumping Jacks 45	Jumping Jacks 45	Jumping Jacks 45	Jumping Jacks 45	Jumping Jacks 45
Running in Place 60 sec.	Running in Place 60 sec.	Running in Place 60 sec.	Running in Place 60 sec.	Running in Place 60 sec.
Half Jumping Jacks 45	Half Jumping Jacks 45	Half Jumping Jacks 45	Half Jumping Jacks 45	Half Jumping Jacks 45
60–90 sec. Rest	60–90 sec. Rest	60–90 sec. Rest	60–90 sec. Rest	60–90 sec. Rest
STRETCHES	**STRETCHES**	**LEGS**	**STRETCHES**	**STRETCHES**
Bend Overs	Chest	Walking Lunges 40 yds. (5x)	Chest	Bend Overs
Cross Overs	Lat	High Knees 40 yds. (5x)	Lat	Cross Overs
Inner Thigh	Shoulders	Frog Hops 40 yds. (5x)	Shoulders	Inner Thigh
Forward Lunge	Tricep	Star Hops 22	Tricep	Forward Lunge
Side & Oblique	Partner	Mountain Climbers 30	Partner	Side & Oblique
Hurdler	Arm Rotation	**SPRINTS**	Arm Rotation	Hurdler
Butterfly	60–90 sec. Rest	Basic Sprints (Optional)	60–90 sec. Rest	Butterfly
ITB	**UPPER BODY**	3 Sets of Cones	**UPPER BODY**	ITB
Thigh	Neck Rotations 40	First Set — 50%	Neck Rotations 40	Thigh
Calf	Back Contractions 40	Second Set — 75%	Back Contractions 40	Calf
60–90 sec. Rest	Swimmer Exercise 40	Third Set — 100%	Swimmer Exercise 40	60–90 sec. Rest
LEGS	Back Lifts 20	20 Sets	Back Lifts 20	**LEGS**
Lunges 45	60–90 sec. Rest		60–90 sec. Rest	Lunges 45
Squats 60	**PULL-UPS**		**PULL-UPS**	Squats 60
Fire Hydrants 40 (Each Side)	Regular 2-4-6-8-10-12-14 ⬇		Regular 2-4-6-8-10-12-14 ⬇	Fire Hydrants 40 (Each Side)
Mountain Climber 30	Close Grip 2-4-6-8-10-12 ⬇		Close Grip 2-4-6-8-10-12 ⬇	Mountain Climber 30
The Wall 3:00 min.	Reverse 2-4-6-8-10-12 ⬇		Reverse 2-4-6-8-10-12 ⬇	The Wall 3:00 min.
60–90 sec. Rest	Commandos 2-4-6-8-6-4-2		Commandos 2-4-6-8-6-4-2	60–90 sec. Rest
CALVES	Behind the Neck 2-4-6-8-6-4-2		Behind the Neck 2-4-6-8-6-4-2	**CALVES**
Straight (Regular) 100	60–90 sec. Rest		60–90 sec. Rest	Straight (Regular) 100
Toe to Toe 100	**BAR DIPS**		**BAR DIPS**	Toe to Toe 100
Heel to Heel 100	Regular 20		Regular 20	Heel to Heel 100
60–90 sec. Rest	60–90 sec. Rest		60–90 sec. Rest	60–90 sec. Rest
ABDOMINALS	**PUSH-UPS**	**ABDOMINALS**	**PUSH-UPS**	**ABDOMINALS**
Hand to Toes 50	Reg. 12-14-16-18-20-22-24 ⬇	Clockwork 50-45-40	Reg. 12-14-16-18-20-22-24 ⬇	Hand to Toes 50
X Sit-Ups 50	Diamond 2-4-6-8-10-12 ⬇	Hanging Knee Up 50	Diamond 2-4-6-8-10-12 ⬇	X Sit-Ups 50
Crunches 50	Dive Bombers 4-6-8-10-12 ⬇	Hanging Side Sit-Up 25	Dive Bombers 4-6-8-10-12 ⬇	Crunches 50
Side Sit-Ups 50	8 Count Body Builders 20	Hand to Toe (Short) 50	8 Count Body Builders 20	Side Sit-Ups 50
Obliques 50	Take "After" Supplements	Crunches (Short) 50	Take "After" Supplements	Obliques 50
Flutter Kicks 50	Drink 16 oz. of water	Side Sit-Up (Short) 50	Drink 16 oz. of water	Flutter Kicks 50
Reverse Crunches 50		Obliques (Short) 50		Reverse Crunches 50
Knee Bends 50		Atomic 40		Knee Bends 50
Chest Roll 50		Take "After" Supplements		Chest Roll 50
Take "After" Supplements		Drink 16 oz. of water		Take "After" Supplements
Drink 16 oz. of water				Drink 16 oz. of water

MEALS 1 2 3 4 5 **WATER** 1 2 3 4 5 6 7 8

SUPPLEMENTS

Before [3] Electrolyte™ [1] Energy Plus™ **After** [3] Recover™ [2] Restore™

(Meals/Water/Supplements blocks repeated identically for Monday, Tuesday, Wednesday, Thursday, and Friday.)

WEEK 4   ADVANCED LEVEL

✓ MONDAY / /	✓ TUESDAY / /	✓ WEDNESDAY / /	✓ THURSDAY / /	✓ FRIDAY / /
Take "Before" Supplements	Take "Before" Supplements	Take "Before" Supplements	Take "Before" Supplements	Take "Before" Supplements
Drink 16 oz. of water	Drink 16 oz. of water	Drink 16 oz. of water	Drink 16 oz. of water	Drink 16 oz. of water
WARM-UPS	**WARM-UPS**	**WARM-UPS**	**WARM-UPS**	**WARM-UPS**
Jumping Jacks 45	Jumping Jacks 45	Jumping Jacks 45	Jumping Jacks 45	Jumping Jacks 45
Running in Place 60 sec.	Running in Place 60 sec.	Running in Place 60 sec.	Running in Place 60 sec.	Running in Place 60 sec.
Half Jumping Jacks 45	Half Jumping Jacks 45	Half Jumping Jacks 45	Half Jumping Jacks 45	Half Jumping Jacks 45
60–90 sec. Rest	60–90 sec. Rest	60–90 sec. Rest	60–90 sec. Rest	60–90 sec. Rest
STRETCHES	**STRETCHES**	**LEGS**	**STRETCHES**	**STRETCHES**
Bend Overs	Chest	Walking Lunges 40 yds. (5x)	Chest	Bend Overs
Cross Overs	Lat	High Knees 40 yds. (5x)	Lat	Cross Overs
Inner Thigh	Shoulders	Frog Hops 40 yds. (5x)	Shoulders	Inner Thigh
Forward Lunge	Tricep	Star Hops 22	Tricep	Forward Lunge
Side & Oblique	Partner	Mountain Climbers 30	Partner	Side & Oblique
Hurdler	Arm Rotation	**SPRINTS**	Arm Rotation	Hurdler
Butterfly	60–90 sec. Rest	Intervals (Optional)	60–90 sec. Rest	Butterfly
ITB	**UPPER BODY**	8 Laps = 3200 yds.	**UPPER BODY**	ITB
Thigh	Neck Rotations 40		Neck Rotations 40	Thigh
Calf	Back Contractions 40		Back Contractions 40	Calf
60–90 sec. Rest	Swimmer Exercise 40		Swimmer Exercise 40	60–90 sec. Rest
LEGS	Back Lifts 20		Back Lifts 20	**LEGS**
Lunges 45	60–90 sec. Rest		60–90 sec. Rest	Lunges 45
Squats 60	**PULL-UPS**		**PULL-UPS**	Squats 60
Fire Hydrants 40 (Each Side)	Regular 2-4-6-8-10-12-14 ⬇		Regular 2-4-6-8-10-12-14 ⬇	Fire Hydrants 40 (Each Side)
Mountain Climber 30	Close Grip 2-4-6-8-10-12 ⬇		Close Grip 2-4-6-8-10-12 ⬇	Mountain Climber 30
The Wall 3:00 min.	Reverse 2-4-6-8-10-12 ⬇		Reverse 2-4-6-8-10-12 ⬇	The Wall 3:00 min.
60–90 sec. Rest	Commandos 2-4-6-8-6-4-2		Commandos 2-4-6-8-6-4-2	60–90 sec. Rest
CALVES	Behind the Neck 2-4-6-8-6-4-2		Behind the Neck 2-4-6-8-6-4-2	**CALVES**
Straight (Regular) 100	60–90 sec. Rest		60–90 sec. Rest	Straight (Regular) 100
Toe to Toe 100	**BAR DIPS**		**BAR DIPS**	Toe to Toe 100
Heel to Heel 100	Regular 20		Regular 20	Heel to Heel 100
60–90 sec. Rest	60–90 sec. Rest		60–90 sec. Rest	60–90 sec. Rest
ABDOMINALS	**PUSH-UPS**		**PUSH-UPS**	**ABDOMINALS**
Hand to Toes 50	Reg. 12-14-16-18-20-22-24 ⬇	**ABDOMINALS**	Reg. 12-14-16-18-20-22-24 ⬇	Hand to Toes 50
X Sit-Ups 50	Diamond 2-4-6-8-10-12 ⬇	Clockwork 50-45-40	Diamond 2-4-6-8-10-12 ⬇	X Sit-Ups 50
Crunches 50	Dive Bombers 4-6-8-10-12 ⬇	Hanging Knee Up 50	Dive Bombers 4-6-8-10-12 ⬇	Crunches 50
Side Sit-Ups 50	8 Count Body Builders 20	Hanging Side Sit-Up 25	8 Count Body Builders 20	Side Sit-Ups 50
Obliques 50	Take "After" Supplements	Hand to Toe (Short) 50	Take "After" Supplements	Obliques 50
Flutter Kicks 50	Drink 16 oz. of water	Crunches (Short) 50	Drink 16 oz. of water	Flutter Kicks 50
Reverse Crunches 50		Side Sit-Up (Short) 50		Reverse Crunches 50
Knee Bends 50		Obliques (Short) 50		Knee Bends 50
Chest Roll 50		Atomic 40		Chest Roll 50
Take "After" Supplements		Take "After" Supplements		Take "After" Supplements
Drink 16 oz. of water		Drink 16 oz. of water		Drink 16 oz. of water

MEALS	WATER	MEALS	WATER	MEALS	WATER	MEALS	WATER	MEALS	WATER
1 2 3 4 / 5	1 2 3 4 / 5 6 7 8	1 2 3 4 / 5	1 2 3 4 / 5 6 7 8	1 2 3 4 / 5	1 2 3 4 / 5 6 7 8	1 2 3 4 / 5	1 2 3 4 / 5 6 7 8	1 2 3 4 / 5	1 2 3 4 / 5 6 7 8

SUPPLEMENTS

Before	After	Before	After	Before	After	Before	After	Before	After
3 Electrolyte™ / **1** Energy Plus™	**3** Recover™ / **2** Restore™	**3** Electrolyte™ / **1** Energy Plus™	**3** Recover™ / **2** Restore™	**3** Electrolyte™ / **1** Energy Plus™	**3** Recover™ / **2** Restore™	**3** Electrolyte™ / **1** Energy Plus™	**3** Recover™ / **2** Restore™	**3** Electrolyte™ / **1** Energy Plus™	**3** Recover™ / **2** Restore™

WEEK 5 — ADVANCED LEVEL

✓ MONDAY / /	✓ TUESDAY / /	✓ WEDNESDAY / /	✓ THURSDAY / /	✓ FRIDAY / /
Take "Before" Supplements	Take "Before" Supplements	Take "Before" Supplements	Take "Before" Supplements	Take "Before" Supplements
Drink 16 oz. of water	Drink 16 oz. of water	Drink 16 oz. of water	Drink 16 oz. of water	Drink 16 oz. of water
WARM-UPS	**WARM-UPS**	**WARM-UPS**	**WARM-UPS**	**WARM-UPS**
Jumping Jacks 45	Jumping Jacks 45	Jumping Jacks 45	Jumping Jacks 45	Jumping Jacks 45
Running in Place 60 sec.	Running in Place 60 sec.	Running in Place 60 sec.	Running in Place 60 sec.	Running in Place 60 sec.
Half Jumping Jacks 45	Half Jumping Jacks 45	Half Jumping Jacks 45	Half Jumping Jacks 45	Half Jumping Jacks 45
60–90 sec. Rest	60–90 sec. Rest	60–90 sec. Rest	60–90 sec. Rest	60–90 sec. Rest
STRETCHES	**STRETCHES**	**LEGS**	**STRETCHES**	**STRETCHES**
Bend Overs	Chest	Walking Lunges 40 yds. (5x)	Chest	Bend Overs
Cross Overs	Lat	High Knees 40 yds. (5x)	Lat	Cross Overs
Inner Thigh	Shoulders	Frog Hops 40 yds. (5x)	Shoulders	Inner Thigh
Forward Lunge	Tricep	Star Hops 22	Tricep	Forward Lunge
Side & Oblique	Partner	Mountain Climbers 30	Partner	Side & Oblique
Hurdler	Arm Rotation	**SPRINTS**	Arm Rotation	Hurdler
Butterfly	60–90 sec. Rest	Basic Sprints (Optional)	60–90 sec. Rest	Butterfly
ITB	**TIMED INTERVALS**	3 Sets of Cones	**UPPER BODY**	ITB
Thigh	**UPPER BODY**	First Set — 50%	Neck Rotations 45	Thigh
Calf	Neck Rotations 90 sec.	Second Set — 75%	Back Contractions 45	Calf
60–90 sec. Rest	Back Contractions 90 sec.	Third Set — 100%	Swimmer Exercise 45	**TIMED INTERVALS**
LEGS	Swimmer Exercise 90 sec.	21 Sets	Back Lifts 25	**LEGS**
Lunges 47	Back Lifts 90 sec.		60–90 sec. Rest	Lunges 90 sec.
Squats 62	60–90 sec. Rest		**PULL-UPS**	Squats 90 sec.
Fire Hydrants 43 (Each Side)	**PULL-UPS**		Regular 2-4-6-8-10-12-14-16 ↓	Fire Hydrants 90 sec. (Each Side)
Mountain Climber 33	Regular 90 sec.		Close Grip 2-4-6-8-10-12 ↓	Mountain Climber 90 sec.
The Wall 3:15 min.	Close Grip 90 sec.		Reverse 2-4-6-8-10-12 ↓	The Wall 3:30 min.
60–90 sec. Rest	Reverse 90 sec.		Commandos 2-4-6-8-10 ↓	60–90 sec. Rest
CALVES	Commandos 90 sec.		Behind the Neck 2-4-6-8-10 ↓	**CALVES**
Straight (Regular) 120	Behind the Neck 90 sec.		60–90 sec. Rest	Straight (Regular) 90 sec.
Toe to Toe 120	60–90 sec. Rest		**BAR DIPS**	Toe to Toe 90 sec.
Heel to Heel 120	**BAR DIPS**		Regular 23	Heel to Heel 90 sec.
60–90 sec. Rest	Regular 90 sec.		60–90 sec. Rest	60–90 sec. Rest
ABDOMINALS	60–90 sec. Rest	**ABDOMINALS**	**PUSH-UPS**	**ABDOMINALS**
Hand to Toes 55	**PUSH-UPS**	Clockwork 55-50-45	Reg. 12-14-16-18-20-22-24-26 ↓	Hand to Toes 90 sec.
X Sit-Ups 55	Regular 90 sec.	Hanging Knee Up 55	Diamond 2-4-6-8-10-12-14 ↓	X Sit-Ups 90 sec.
Crunches 55	Diamond 90 sec.	Hanging Side Sit-Up 22	Dive Bombers 4-6-8-10-12-14 ↓	Crunches 90 sec.
Side Sit-Ups 55	Dive Bombers 90 sec.	Hand to Toe (Short) 55	8 Count Body Builders 22	Side Sit-Ups 90 sec.
Obliques 55	8 Count Body Builders 90 sec.	Crunches (Short) 55	Take "After" Supplements	Obliques 90 sec.
Flutter Kicks 55	Take "After" Supplements	Side Sit-Up (Short) 55	Drink 16 oz. of water	Flutter Kicks 90 sec.
Reverse Crunches 55	Drink 16 oz. of water	Obliques (Short) 55		Reverse Crunches 90 sec.
Knee Bends 55		Atomic 45		Knee Bends 90 sec.
Chest Roll 55		Take "After" Supplements		Chest Roll 90 sec.
Take "After" Supplements		Drink 16 oz. of water		Take "After" Supplements
Drink 16 oz. of water				Drink 1 quart of water

MONDAY

MEALS: 1 2 3 4 5 — WATER: 1 2 3 4 5 6 7 8

SUPPLEMENTS
Before: 3 Electrolyte™ / 1 Energy Plus™
After: 3 Recover™ / 2 Restore™

TUESDAY

MEALS: 1 2 3 4 5 — WATER: 1 2 3 4 5 6 7 8

SUPPLEMENTS
Before: 3 Electrolyte™ / 1 Energy Plus™
After: 3 Recover™ / 2 Restore™

WEDNESDAY

MEALS: 1 2 3 4 5 — WATER: 1 2 3 4 5 6 7 8

SUPPLEMENTS
Before: 3 Electrolyte™ / 1 Energy Plus™
After: 3 Recover™ / 2 Restore™

THURSDAY

MEALS: 1 2 3 4 5 — WATER: 1 2 3 4 5 6 7 8

SUPPLEMENTS
Before: 3 Electrolyte™ / 1 Energy Plus™
After: 3 Recover™ / 2 Restore™

FRIDAY

MEALS: 1 2 3 4 5 — WATER: 1 2 3 4 5 6 7 8

SUPPLEMENTS
Before: 3 Electrolyte™ / 1 Energy Plus™
After: 3 Recover™ / 2 Restore™

WEEK 6　　ADVANCED LEVEL

✓ MONDAY / /	✓ TUESDAY / /	✓ WEDNESDAY / /	✓ THURSDAY / /	✓ FRIDAY / /
Take "Before" Supplements	Take "Before" Supplements	Take "Before" Supplements	Take "Before" Supplements	Take "Before" Supplements
Drink 16 oz. of water	Drink 16 oz. of water	Drink 16 oz. of water	Drink 16 oz. of water	Drink 16 oz. of water
WARM-UPS	**WARM-UPS**	**WARM-UPS**	**WARM-UPS**	**WARM-UPS**
Jumping Jacks 45	Jumping Jacks 45	Jumping Jacks 45	Jumping Jacks 45	Jumping Jacks 45
Running in Place 60 sec.	Running in Place 60 sec.	Running in Place 60 sec.	Running in Place 60 sec.	Running in Place 60 sec.
Half Jumping Jacks 45	Half Jumping Jacks 45	Half Jumping Jacks 45	Half Jumping Jacks 45	Half Jumping Jacks 45
60–90 sec. Rest	60–90 sec. Rest	60–90 sec. Rest	60–90 sec. Rest	60–90 sec. Rest
STRETCHES	**STRETCHES**	**LEGS**	**STRETCHES**	**STRETCHES**
Bend Overs	Chest	Walking Lunges 40 yds. (5x)	Chest	Bend Overs
Cross Overs	Lat	High Knees 40 yds. (5x)	Lat	Cross Overs
Inner Thigh	Shoulders	Frog Hops 40 yds. (5x)	Shoulders	Inner Thigh
Forward Lunge	Tricep	Star Hops 22	Tricep	Forward Lunge
Side & Oblique	Partner	Mountain Climbers 30	Partner	Side & Oblique
Hurdler	Arm Rotation	**SPRINTS**	Arm Rotation	Hurdler
Butterfly	60–90 sec. Rest	Intervals (Optional)	60–90 sec. Rest	Butterfly
ITB	**UPPER BODY**	9 Laps = 3600 yds.	**UPPER BODY**	ITB
Thigh	Neck Rotations 45		Neck Rotations 45	Thigh
Calf	Back Contractions 45		Back Contractions 45	Calf
60–90 sec. Rest	Swimmer Exercise 45		Swimmer Exercise 45	60–90 sec. Rest
LEGS	Back Lifts 25		Back Lifts 25	**LEGS**
Lunges 47	60–90 sec. Rest		60–90 sec. Rest	Lunges 47
Squats 62	**PULL-UPS**		**PULL-UPS**	Squats 62
Fire Hydrants 43 (Each Side)	Regular 2-4-6-8-10-12-14-16 ⬇		Regular 2-4-6-8-10-12-14-16 ⬇	Fire Hydrants 43 (Each Side)
Mountain Climber 33	Close Grip 2-4-6-8-10-12 ⬇		Close Grip 2-4-6-8-10-12 ⬇	Mountain Climber 33
The Wall 3:15 min.	Reverse 2-4-6-8-10-12 ⬇		Reverse 2-4-6-8-10-12 ⬇	The Wall 3:15 min.
60–90 sec. Rest	Commandos 2-4-6-8-10 ⬇		Commandos 2-4-6-8-10 ⬇	60–90 sec. Rest
CALVES	Behind the Neck 2-4-6-8-10 ⬇		Behind the Neck 2-4-6-8-10 ⬇	**CALVES**
Straight (Regular) 120	60–90 sec. Rest		60–90 sec. Rest	Straight (Regular) 120
Toe to Toe 120	**BAR DIPS**		**BAR DIPS**	Toe to Toe 120
Heel to Heel 120	Regular 23		Regular 23	Heel to Heel 120
60–90 sec. Rest	60–90 sec. Rest		60–90 sec. Rest	60–90 sec. Rest
ABDOMINALS	**PUSH-UPS**		**PUSH-UPS**	**ABDOMINALS**
Hand to Toes 55	Reg. 12-14-16-18-20-22-24-26 ⬇	**ABDOMINALS**	Reg. 12-14-16-18-20-22-24-26 ⬇	Hand to Toes 55
X Sit-Ups 55	Diamond 2-4-6-8-10-12-14 ⬇	Clockwork 55-50-45	Diamond 2-4-6-8-10-12-14 ⬇	X Sit-Ups 55
Crunches 55	Dive Bombers 2-4-6-8-10-12-14 ⬇	Hanging Knee Up 55	Dive Bombers 2-4-6-8-10-12-14 ⬇	Crunches 55
Side Sit-Ups 55	8 Count Body Builders 22	Hanging Side Sit-Up 22	8 Count Body Builders 22	Side Sit-Ups 55
Obliques 55	Take "After" Supplements	Hand to Toe (Short) 55	Take "After" Supplements	Obliques 55
Flutter Kicks 55	Drink 16 oz. of water	Crunches (Short) 55	Drink 16 oz. of water	Flutter Kicks 55
Reverse Crunches 55		Side Sit-Up (Short) 55		Reverse Crunches 55
Knee Bends 55		Obliques (Short) 55		Knee Bends 55
Chest Roll 55		Atomic 45		Chest Roll 55
Take "After" Supplements		Take "After" Supplements		Take "After" Supplements
Drink 16 oz. of water		Drink 16 oz. of water		Drink 16 oz. of water

MEALS 1 2 3 4 5 　**WATER** 1 2 3 4 5 6 7 8
SUPPLEMENTS
Before: 3 Electrolyte™　1 Energy Plus™
After: 3 Recover™　2 Restore™

MEALS 1 2 3 4 5 　**WATER** 1 2 3 4 5 6 7 8
SUPPLEMENTS
Before: 3 Electrolyte™　1 Energy Plus™
After: 3 Recover™　2 Restore™

MEALS 1 2 3 4 5 　**WATER** 1 2 3 4 5 6 7 8
SUPPLEMENTS
Before: 3 Electrolyte™　1 Energy Plus™
After: 3 Recover™　2 Restore™

MEALS 1 2 3 4 5 　**WATER** 1 2 3 4 5 6 7 8
SUPPLEMENTS
Before: 3 Electrolyte™　1 Energy Plus™
After: 3 Recover™　2 Restore™

MEALS 1 2 3 4 5 　**WATER** 1 2 3 4 5 6 7 8
SUPPLEMENTS
Before: 3 Electrolyte™　1 Energy Plus™
After: 3 Recover™　2 Restore™

WEEK 7   ADVANCED LEVEL

✓ MONDAY / /	✓ TUESDAY / /	✓ WEDNESDAY / /	✓ THURSDAY / /	✓ FRIDAY / /
Take "Before" Supplements	Take "Before" Supplements	Take "Before" Supplements	Take "Before" Supplements	Take "Before" Supplements
Drink 16 oz. of water	Drink 16 oz. of water	Drink 16 oz. of water	Drink 16 oz. of water	Drink 16 oz. of water
WARM-UPS	**WARM-UPS**	**WARM-UPS**	**WARM-UPS**	**WARM-UPS**
Jumping Jacks 45	Jumping Jacks 45	Jumping Jacks 45	Jumping Jacks 45	Jumping Jacks 45
Running in Place 60 sec.	Running in Place 60 sec.	Running in Place 60 sec.	Running in Place 60 sec.	Running in Place 60 sec.
Half Jumping Jacks 45	Half Jumping Jacks 45	Half Jumping Jacks 45	Half Jumping Jacks 45	Half Jumping Jacks 45
60–90 sec. Rest	60–90 sec. Rest	60–90 sec. Rest	60–90 sec. Rest	60–90 sec. Rest
STRETCHES	**STRETCHES**	**LEGS**	**STRETCHES**	**STRETCHES**
Bend Overs	Chest	Walking Lunges 40 yds. (5x)	Chest	Bend Overs
Cross Overs	Lat	High Knees 40 yds. (5x)	Lat	Cross Overs
Inner Thigh	Shoulders	Frog Hops 40 yds. (5x)	Shoulders	Inner Thigh
Forward Lunge	Tricep	Star Hops 22	Tricep	Forward Lunge
Side & Oblique	Partner	Mountain Climbers 30	Partner	Side & Oblique
Hurdler	Arm Rotation	**SPRINTS**	Arm Rotation	Hurdler
Butterfly	60–90 sec. Rest	Basic Sprints (Optional)	60–90 sec. Rest	Butterfly
ITB	**UPPER BODY**	3 Sets of Cones	**UPPER BODY**	ITB
Thigh	Neck Rotations 45	First Set — 50%	Neck Rotations 45	Thigh
Calf	Back Contractions 45	Second Set — 75%	Back Contractions 45	Calf
60–90 sec. Rest	Swimmer Exercise 45	Third Set — 100%	Swimmer Exercise 45	60–90 sec. Rest
LEGS	Back Lifts 25	22 Sets	Back Lifts 25	**LEGS**
Lunges 47	60–90 sec. Rest		60–90 sec. Rest	Lunges 47
Squats 62	**PULL-UPS**		**PULL-UPS**	Squats 62
Fire Hydrants 43 (Each Side)	Regular 2-4-6-8-10-12-14-16 ⬇		Regular 2-4-6-8-10-12-14-16 ⬇	Fire Hydrants 43 (Each Side)
Mountain Climber 33	Close Grip 2-4-6-8-10-12 ⬇		Close Grip 2-4-6-8-10-12 ⬇	Mountain Climber 33
The Wall 3:15 min.	Reverse 2-4-6-8-10-12 ⬇		Reverse 2-4-6-8-10-12 ⬇	The Wall 3:15 min.
60–90 sec. Rest	Commandos 2-4-6-8-10 ⬇		Commandos 2-4-6-8-10 ⬇	60–90 sec. Rest
CALVES	Behind the Neck 2-4-6-8-10 ⬇		Behind the Neck 2-4-6-8-10 ⬇	**CALVES**
Straight (Regular) 120	60–90 sec. Rest		60–90 sec. Rest	Straight (Regular) 120
Toe to Toe 120	**BAR DIPS**		**BAR DIPS**	Toe to Toe 120
Heel to Heel 120	Regular 23		Regular 23	Heel to Heel 120
60–90 sec. Rest	60–90 sec. Rest		60–90 sec. Rest	60–90 sec. Rest
ABDOMINALS	**PUSH-UPS**	**ABDOMINALS**	**PUSH-UPS**	**ABDOMINALS**
Hand to Toes 55	Reg. 12-14-16-18-20-22-24-26 ⬇	Clockwork 55-50-45	Reg. 12-14-16-18-20-22-24-26 ⬇	Hand to Toes 55
X Sit-Ups 55	Diamond 2-4-6-8-10-12-14 ⬇	Hanging Knee Up 55	Diamond 2-4-6-8-10-12-14 ⬇	X Sit-Ups 55
Crunches 55	Dive Bombers 2-4-6-8-10-12-14 ⬇	Hanging Side Sit-Up 22	Dive Bombers 2-4-6-8-10-12-14 ⬇	Crunches 55
Side Sit-Ups 55	8 Count Body Builders 22	Hand to Toe (Short) 55	8 Count Body Builders 22	Side Sit-Ups 55
Obliques 55	Take "After" Supplements	Crunches (Short) 55	Take "After" Supplements	Obliques 55
Flutter Kicks 55	Drink 16 oz. of water	Side Sit-Up (Short) 55	Drink 16 oz. of water	Flutter Kicks 55
Reverse Crunches 55		Obliques (Short) 55		Reverse Crunches 55
Knee Bends 55		Atomic 45		Knee Bends 55
Chest Roll 55		Take "After" Supplements		Chest Roll 55
Take "After" Supplements		Drink 16 oz. of water		Take "After" Supplements
Drink 16 oz. of water				Drink 16 oz. of water

MEALS / WATER	MEALS / WATER	MEALS / WATER	MEALS / WATER	MEALS / WATER
MEALS 1 2 3 4 / 5 WATER 1 2 3 4 / 5 6 7 8	MEALS 1 2 3 4 / 5 WATER 1 2 3 4 / 5 6 7 8	MEALS 1 2 3 4 / 5 WATER 1 2 3 4 / 5 6 7 8	MEALS 1 2 3 4 / 5 WATER 1 2 3 4 / 5 6 7 8	MEALS 1 2 3 4 / 5 WATER 1 2 3 4 / 5 6 7 8
SUPPLEMENTS	**SUPPLEMENTS**	**SUPPLEMENTS**	**SUPPLEMENTS**	**SUPPLEMENTS**
Before: 3 Electrolyte™ / 1 Energy Plus™ — After: 3 Recover™ / 2 Restore™	Before: 3 Electrolyte™ / 1 Energy Plus™ — After: 3 Recover™ / 2 Restore™	Before: 3 Electrolyte™ / 1 Energy Plus™ — After: 3 Recover™ / 2 Restore™	Before: 3 Electrolyte™ / 1 Energy Plus™ — After: 3 Recover™ / 2 Restore™	Before: 3 Electrolyte™ / 1 Energy Plus™ — After: 3 Recover™ / 2 Restore™

WEEK 8 — ADVANCED LEVEL

✓ MONDAY / /	✓ TUESDAY / /	✓ WEDNESDAY / /	✓ THURSDAY / /	✓ FRIDAY / /
Take "Before" Supplements	Take "Before" Supplements	Take "Before" Supplements	Take "Before" Supplements	Take "Before" Supplements
Drink 16 oz. of water	Drink 16 oz. of water	Drink 16 oz. of water	Drink 16 oz. of water	Drink 16 oz. of water
WARM-UPS	**WARM-UPS**	**WARM-UPS**	**WARM-UPS**	**WARM-UPS**
Jumping Jacks 45	Jumping Jacks 45	Jumping Jacks 45	Jumping Jacks 45	Jumping Jacks 45
Running in Place 60 sec.	Running in Place 60 sec.	Running in Place 60 sec.	Running in Place 60 sec.	Running in Place 60 sec.
Half Jumping Jacks 45	Half Jumping Jacks 45	Half Jumping Jacks 45	Half Jumping Jacks 45	Half Jumping Jacks 45
60–90 sec. Rest	60–90 sec. Rest	60–90 sec. Rest	60–90 sec. Rest	60–90 sec. Rest
STRETCHES	**STRETCHES**	**LEGS**	**STRETCHES**	**STRETCHES**
Bend Overs	Chest	Walking Lunges 40 yds. (5x)	Chest	Bend Overs
Cross Overs	Lat	High Knees 40 yds. (5x)	Lat	Cross Overs
Inner Thigh	Shoulders	Frog Hops 40 yds. (5x)	Shoulders	Inner Thigh
Forward Lunge	Tricep	Star Hops 24	Tricep	Forward Lunge
Side & Oblique	Partner	Mountain Climbers 30	Partner	Side & Oblique
Hurdler	Arm Rotation	**SPRINTS**	Arm Rotation	Hurdler
Butterfly	60–90 sec. Rest	Intervals (Optional)	60–90 sec. Rest	Butterfly
ITB	***TIMED INTERVALS***	10 Laps = 4000 yds.	***CIRCUIT—***	ITB
Thigh	**UPPER BODY**		***UPPER BODY***	Thigh
Calf	Neck Rotations 90 sec.		**SET 1**	Calf
60–90 sec. Rest	Back Contractions 90 sec.		Regular Pull-Ups 25	***TIMED INTERVALS***
CIRCUIT—	Swimmer Exercise 90 sec.		Bar Dips 35	**LEGS**
LEGS	Back Lifts 90 sec.		Regular Push-Ups 70	Lunges 90 sec.
SET 1	60–90 sec. Rest		**SET 2**	Squats 90 sec.
The Wall 3:30 min.	**PULL-UPS**		Close Grip Pull-Ups 25	Fire Hydrants 90 sec. (Each Side)
Frog Hops 40 yds. (6x)	Regular 90 sec.		Bar Dips 35	Mountain Climber 90 sec.
Hand to Toe 50	Close Grip 90 sec.		Diamond Push-Ups 45	The Wall 3:45 min.
SET 2	Reverse 90 sec.		**SET 3**	60–90 sec. Rest
Walking Lunges 40 yds. (6x)	Commandos 90 sec.		Reverse Grip Pull-Ups 25	**CALVES**
Star Hops 25	Behind the Neck 90 sec.		Bar Dips 35	Straight (Regular) 90 sec.
Side Sit-Ups 50	60–90 sec. Rest		Dive Bombers 45	Toe to Toe 90 sec.
SET 3	**BAR DIPS**		**SET 4**	Heel to Heel 90 sec.
Mountain Climbers 25	Regular 90 sec.		Behind the Neck Pull-Ups 20	60–90 sec. Rest
Regular Calf Raises 100	60–90 sec. Rest		Bar Dips 35	**ABDOMINALS**
Knee Bends 50	**PUSH-UPS**	**ABDOMINALS**	Regular Push-Ups 70	Hand to Toes 90 sec.
SET 4	Regular 90 sec.	Clockwork 55-50-45	Take "After" Supplements	X Sit-Ups 90 sec.
Fire Hydrants 50 (Each Side)	Diamond 90 sec.	Hanging Knee Up 55	Drink 16 oz. of water	Crunches 90 sec.
Toe to Toe Calf Raises 100	Dive Bombers 90 sec.	Hanging Side Sit-Up 22		Side Sit-Ups 90 sec.
Crunches 50	8 Count Body Builders 90 sec.	Hand to Toe (Short) 55		Obliques 90 sec.
SET 5	Take "After" Supplements	Crunches (Short) 55		Flutter Kicks 90 sec.
Heel to Heel Calf Raises 100	Drink 16 oz. of water	Side Sit-Up (Short) 55		Reverse Crunches 90 sec.
Knee Roll Ups 50		Obliques (Short) 55		Knee Bends 90 sec.
Take "After" Supplements		Atomic 45		Chest Roll 90 sec.
Drink 16 oz. of water		Take "After" Supplements		Take "After" Supplements
		Drink 16 oz. of water		Drink 1 quart of water

	MONDAY	TUESDAY	WEDNESDAY	THURSDAY	FRIDAY
MEALS	1 2 3 4 5	1 2 3 4 5	1 2 3 4 5	1 2 3 4 5	1 2 3 4 5
WATER	1 2 3 4 5 6 7 8	1 2 3 4 5 6 7 8	1 2 3 4 5 6 7 8	1 2 3 4 5 6 7 8	1 2 3 4 5 6 7 8

SUPPLEMENTS

	Before	After	Before	After	Before	After	Before	After	Before	After
	3 Electrolyte™	3 Recover™	3 Electrolyte™	3 Recover™	3 Electrolyte™	3 Recover™	3 Electrolyte™	3 Recover™	3 Electrolyte™	3 Recover™
	1 Energy Plus™	2 Restore™	1 Energy Plus™	2 Restore™	1 Energy Plus™	2 Restore™	1 Energy Plus™	2 Restore™	1 Energy Plus™	2 Restore™

✓ MONDAY / /	✓ TUESDAY / /	✓ WEDNESDAY / /	✓ THURSDAY / /	✓ FRIDAY / /
Take "Before" Supplements	Take "Before" Supplements	Take "Before" Supplements	Take "Before" Supplements	Take "Before" Supplements
Drink 16 oz. of water	Drink 16 oz. of water	Drink 16 oz. of water	Drink 16 oz. of water	Drink 16 oz. of water
WARM-UPS	**WARM-UPS**	**WARM-UPS**	**WARM-UPS**	**WARM-UPS**
Jumping Jacks 45	Jumping Jacks 45	Jumping Jacks 45	Jumping Jacks 45	Jumping Jacks 45
Running in Place 60 sec.	Running in Place 60 sec.	Running in Place 60 sec.	Running in Place 60 sec.	Running in Place 60 sec.
Half Jumping Jacks 45	Half Jumping Jacks 45	Half Jumping Jacks 45	Half Jumping Jacks 45	Half Jumping Jacks 45
60–90 sec. Rest	60–90 sec. Rest	60–90 sec. Rest	60–90 sec. Rest	60–90 sec. Rest
STRETCHES	**STRETCHES**	**LEGS**	**STRETCHES**	**STRETCHES**
Bend Overs	Chest	Walking Lunges 40 yds. (5x)	Chest	Bend Overs
Cross Overs	Lat	High Knees 40 yds. (5x)	Lat	Cross Overs
Inner Thigh	Shoulders	Frog Hops 40 yds. (5x)	Shoulders	Inner Thigh
Forward Lunge	Tricep	Star Hops 25	Tricep	Forward Lunge
Side & Oblique	Partner	Mountain Climbers 32	Partner	Side & Oblique
Hurdler	Arm Rotation	**SPRINTS**	Arm Rotation	Hurdler
Butterfly	60–90 sec. Rest	Basic Sprints (Optional)	60–90 sec. Rest	Butterfly
ITB	**UPPER BODY**	3 Sets of Cones	**UPPER BODY**	ITB
Thigh	Neck Rotations 50	First Set — 50%	Neck Rotations 50	Thigh
Calf	Back Contractions 50	Second Set — 75%	Back Contractions 50	Calf
60–90 sec. Rest	Swimmer Exercise 50	Third Set — 100%	Swimmer Exercise 50	60–90 sec. Rest
LEGS	Back Lifts 30	23 Sets	Back Lifts 30	**LEGS**
Lunges 50	60–90 sec. Rest		60–90 sec. Rest	Lunges 50
Squats 65	**PULL-UPS**		**PULL-UPS**	Squats 65
Fire Hydrants 45 (Each Side)	Regular 4-6-8-10-12-14-16-18 ⬇		Regular 4-6-8-10-12-14-16-18 ⬇	Fire Hydrants 45 (Each Side)
Mountain Climber 35	Close Grip 2-4-6-8-10-12-14 ⬇		Close Grip 2-4-6-8-10-12-14 ⬇	Mountain Climber 35
The Wall 3:30 min.	Reverse 2-4-6-8-10-12-14 ⬇		Reverse 2-4-6-8-10-12-14 ⬇	The Wall 3:30 min.
60–90 sec. Rest	Commandos 2-4-6-8-10-12 ⬇		Commandos 2-4-6-8-10-12 ⬇	60–90 sec. Rest
CALVES	Behind the Neck 2-4-6-8-10-12 ⬇		Behind the Neck 2-4-6-8-10-12 ⬇	**CALVES**
Straight (Regular) 140	60–90 sec. Rest		60–90 sec. Rest	Straight (Regular) 140
Toe to Toe 140	**BAR DIPS**		**BAR DIPS**	Toe to Toe 140
Heel to Heel 140	Regular 25		Regular 25	Heel to Heel 140
60–90 sec. Rest	60–90 sec. Rest		60–90 sec. Rest	60–90 sec. Rest
ABDOMINALS	**PUSH-UPS**		**PUSH-UPS**	**ABDOMINALS**
Hand to Toes 60	Reg. 14-16-18-20-22-24-26-28 ⬇	**ABDOMINALS**	Reg. 14-16-18-20-22-24-26-28 ⬇	Hand to Toes 60
X Sit-Ups 60	Diamond 4-6-8-10-12-14-16 ⬇	Clockwork 60-55-50	Diamond 4-6-8-10-12-14-16 ⬇	X Sit-Ups 60
Crunches 60	Dive Bombers 4-6-8-10-12-14-16 ⬇	Hanging Knee Up 60	Dive Bombers 4-6-8-10-12-14-16 ⬇	Crunches 60
Side Sit-Ups 60	8 Count Body Builders 24	Hanging Side Sit-Up 30	8 Count Body Builders 24	Side Sit-Ups 60
Obliques 60	Take "After" Supplements	Hand to Toe (Short) 60	Take "After" Supplements	Obliques 60
Flutter Kicks 60	Drink 16 oz. of water	Crunches (Short) 60	Drink 16 oz. of water	Flutter Kicks 60
Reverse Crunches 60		Side Sit-Up (Short) 60		Reverse Crunches 60
Knee Bends 60		Obliques (Short) 60		Knee Bends 60
Chest Roll 60		Atomic 50		Chest Roll 60
Take "After" Supplements		Take "After" Supplements		Take "After" Supplements
Drink 16 oz. of water		Drink 16 oz. of water		Drink 16 oz. of water

MONDAY
MEALS: 1 2 3 4 5
WATER: 1 2 3 4 5 6 7 8
SUPPLEMENTS
Before: 3 Electrolyte™ 1 Energy Plus™
After: 3 Recover™ 2 Restore™

TUESDAY
MEALS: 1 2 3 4 5
WATER: 1 2 3 4 5 6 7 8
SUPPLEMENTS
Before: 3 Electrolyte™ 1 Energy Plus™
After: 3 Recover™ 2 Restore™

WEDNESDAY
MEALS: 1 2 3 4 5
WATER: 1 2 3 4 5 6 7 8
SUPPLEMENTS
Before: 3 Electrolyte™ 1 Energy Plus™
After: 3 Recover™ 2 Restore™

THURSDAY
MEALS: 1 2 3 4 5
WATER: 1 2 3 4 5 6 7 8
SUPPLEMENTS
Before: 3 Electrolyte™ 1 Energy Plus™
After: 3 Recover™ 2 Restore™

FRIDAY
MEALS: 1 2 3 4 5
WATER: 1 2 3 4 5 6 7 8
SUPPLEMENTS
Before: 3 Electrolyte™ 1 Energy Plus™
After: 3 Recover™ 2 Restore™

WEEK 10 — ADVANCED LEVEL

✓ MONDAY / /	✓ TUESDAY / /	✓ WEDNESDAY / /	✓ THURSDAY / /	✓ FRIDAY / /
Take "Before" Supplements	Take "Before" Supplements	Take "Before" Supplements	Take "Before" Supplements	Take "Before" Supplements
Drink 16 oz. of water	Drink 16 oz. of water	Drink 16 oz. of water	Drink 16 oz. of water	Drink 16 oz. of water
WARM-UPS	**WARM-UPS**	**WARM-UPS**	**WARM-UPS**	**WARM-UPS**
Jumping Jacks 45	Jumping Jacks 45	Jumping Jacks 45	Jumping Jacks 45	Jumping Jacks 45
Running in Place 60 sec.	Running in Place 60 sec.	Running in Place 60 sec.	Running in Place 60 sec.	Running in Place 60 sec.
Half Jumping Jacks 45	Half Jumping Jacks 45	Half Jumping Jacks 45	Half Jumping Jacks 45	Half Jumping Jacks 45
60–90 sec. Rest	60–90 sec. Rest	60–90 sec. Rest	60–90 sec. Rest	60–90 sec. Rest
STRETCHES	**STRETCHES**	**LEGS**	**STRETCHES**	**STRETCHES**
Bend Overs	Chest	Walking Lunges 40 yds. (5x)	Chest	Bend Overs
Cross Overs	Lat	High Knees 40 yds. (5x)	Lat	Cross Overs
Inner Thigh	Shoulders	Frog Hops 40 yds. (5x)	Shoulders	Inner Thigh
Forward Lunge	Tricep	Star Hops 25	Tricep	Forward Lunge
Side & Oblique	Partner	Mountain Climbers 32	Partner	Side & Oblique
Hurdler	Arm Rotation	**SPRINTS**	Arm Rotation	Hurdler
Butterfly	60–90 sec. Rest	Intervals (Optional)	60–90 sec. Rest	Butterfly
ITB	**UPPER BODY**	11 Laps = 4400 yds.	***BURNOUTS— UPPER BODY***	ITB
Thigh	Neck Rotations 50			Thigh
Calf	Back Contractions 50		**SET 1**	Calf
60–90 sec. Rest	Swimmer Exercise 50		Regular Pull-Ups	60–90 sec. Rest
LEGS	Back Lifts 30		Bar Dips	***BURNOUTS— LEGS***
Lunges 50	60–90 sec. Rest		Regular Push-Ups	
Squats 65	**PULL-UPS**		**SET 2**	**SET 1**
Fire Hydrants 45 (Each Side)	Regular 4-6-8-10-12-14-16-18 ⬇		Close Grip Pull-Ups	The Wall
Mountain Climber 35	Close Grip 2-4-6-8-10-12-14 ⬇		Bar Dips	Frog Hops
The Wall 3:30 min.	Reverse 2-4-6-8-10-12-14 ⬇		Diamond Push-Ups	Hand to Toe
60–90 sec. Rest	Commandos 2-4-6-8-10-12 ⬇		**SET 3**	**SET 2**
CALVES	Behind the Neck 2-4-6-8-10-12 ⬇		Reverse Grip Pull-Ups	Lunges
Straight (Regular) 140	60–90 sec. Rest		Bar Dips	Star Hops
Toe to Toe 140	**BAR DIPS**		Dive Bombers	Side Sit-Ups
Heel to Heel 140	Regular 25		**SET 4**	**SET 3**
60–90 sec. Rest	60–90 sec. Rest		Behind the Neck Pull-Ups	Mountain Climbers
ABDOMINALS	**PUSH-UPS**		Bar Dips	Atomics
Hand to Toes 60	Reg. 14-16-18-20-22-24-26-28 ⬇	**ABDOMINALS**	Regular Push-Ups	Knee Bends
X Sit-Ups 60	Diamond 4-6-8-10-12-14-16 ⬇	Clockwork 60-55-50	**SET 5**	**SET 4**
Crunches 60	Dive Bombers 4-6-8-10-12-14-16 ⬇	Hanging Knee Up 60	Commandos	Fire Hydrants (Each Side)
Side Sit-Ups 60	8 Count Body Builders 24	Hanging Side Sit-Up 30	Bar Dips	High Knees
Obliques 60	Take "After" Supplements	Hand to Toe (Short) 60	Diamond Push-Ups	Crunches
Flutter Kicks 60	Drink 16 oz. of water	Crunches (Short) 60	Take "After" Supplements	**SET 5**
Reverse Crunches 60		Side Sit-Up (Short) 60	Drink 16 oz. of water	Calf Raises
Knee Bends 60		Obliques (Short) 60		Sprints
Chest Roll 60		Atomic 50		Knee Roll Ups
Take "After" Supplements		Take "After" Supplements		Take "After" Supplements
Drink 16 oz. of water		Drink 16 oz. of water		Drink 1 quart of water

MEALS / WATER / SUPPLEMENTS

	MEALS	WATER	SUPPLEMENTS Before	SUPPLEMENTS After
Monday	1 2 3 4 5	1 2 3 4 5 6 7 8	3 Electrolyte™ / 1 Energy Plus™	3 Recover™ / 2 Restore™
Tuesday	1 2 3 4 5	1 2 3 4 5 6 7 8	3 Electrolyte™ / 1 Energy Plus™	3 Recover™ / 2 Restore™
Wednesday	1 2 3 4 5	1 2 3 4 5 6 7 8	3 Electrolyte™ / 1 Energy Plus™	3 Recover™ / 2 Restore™
Thursday	1 2 3 4 5	1 2 3 4 5 6 7 8	3 Electrolyte™ / 1 Energy Plus™	3 Recover™ / 2 Restore™
Friday	1 2 3 4 5	1 2 3 4 5 6 7 8	3 Electrolyte™ / 1 Energy Plus™	3 Recover™ / 2 Restore™

WEEK 11 — ADVANCED LEVEL

✓ MONDAY / /	✓ TUESDAY / /	✓ WEDNESDAY / /	✓ THURSDAY / /	✓ FRIDAY / /
Take "Before" Supplements	Take "Before" Supplements	Take "Before" Supplements	Take "Before" Supplements	Take "Before" Supplements
Drink 16 oz. of water	Drink 16 oz. of water	Drink 16 oz. of water	Drink 16 oz. of water	Drink 16 oz. of water
WARM-UPS	**WARM-UPS**	**WARM-UPS**	**WARM-UPS**	**WARM-UPS**
Jumping Jacks 45	Jumping Jacks 45	Jumping Jacks 45	Jumping Jacks 45	Jumping Jacks 45
Running in Place 60 sec.	Running in Place 60 sec.	Running in Place 60 sec.	Running in Place 60 sec.	Running in Place 60 sec.
Half Jumping Jacks 45	Half Jumping Jacks 45	Half Jumping Jacks 45	Half Jumping Jacks 45	Half Jumping Jacks 45
60–90 sec. Rest	60–90 sec. Rest	60–90 sec. Rest	60–90 sec. Rest	60–90 sec. Rest
STRETCHES	**STRETCHES**	**LEGS**	**STRETCHES**	**STRETCHES**
Bend Overs	Chest	Walking Lunges 40 yds. (5x)	Chest	Bend Overs
Cross Overs	Lat	High Knees 40 yds. (5x)	Lat	Cross Overs
Inner Thigh	Shoulders	Frog Hops 40 yds. (5x)	Shoulders	Inner Thigh
Forward Lunge	Tricep	Star Hops 25	Tricep	Forward Lunge
Side & Oblique	Partner	Mountain Climbers 32	Partner	Side & Oblique
Hurdler	Arm Rotation	**SPRINTS**	Arm Rotation	Hurdler
Butterfly	60–90 sec. Rest	Basic Sprints (Optional)	60–90 sec. Rest	Butterfly
ITB	**UPPER BODY**	3 Sets of Cones	**UPPER BODY**	ITB
Thigh	Neck Rotations 50	First Set — 50%	Neck Rotations 50	Thigh
Calf	Back Contractions 50	Second Set — 75%	Back Contractions 50	Calf
60–90 sec. Rest	Swimmer Exercise 50	Third Set — 100%	Swimmer Exercise 50	60–90 sec. Rest
LEGS	Back Lifts 30	24 Sets	Back Lifts 30	**LEGS**
Lunges 50	60–90 sec. Rest		60–90 sec. Rest	Lunges 50
Squats 65	**PULL-UPS**		**PULL-UPS**	Squats 65
Fire Hydrants 45 (Each Side)	Regular 4-6-8-10-12-14-16-18 ⬇		Regular 4-6-8-10-12-14-16-18 ⬇	Fire Hydrants 45 (Each Side)
Mountain Climber 35	Close Grip 2-4-6-8-10-12-14 ⬇		Close Grip 2-4-6-8-10-12-14 ⬇	Mountain Climber 35
The Wall 3:30 min.	Reverse 2-4-6-8-10-12-14 ⬇		Reverse 2-4-6-8-10-12-14 ⬇	The Wall 3:30 min.
60–90 sec. Rest	Commandos 2-4-6-8-10-12 ⬇		Commandos 2-4-6-8-10-12 ⬇	60–90 sec. Rest
CALVES	Behind the Neck 2-4-6-8-10-12 ⬇		Behind the Neck 2-4-6-8-10-12 ⬇	**CALVES**
Straight (Regular) 140	60–90 sec. Rest		60–90 sec. Rest	Straight (Regular) 140
Toe to Toe 140	**BAR DIPS**		**BAR DIPS**	Toe to Toe 140
Heel to Heel 140	Regular 25		Regular 25	Heel to Heel 140
60–90 sec. Rest	60–90 sec. Rest		60–90 sec. Rest	60–90 sec. Rest
ABDOMINALS	**PUSH-UPS**		**PUSH-UPS**	**ABDOMINALS**
Hand to Toes 60	Reg. 14-16-18-20-22-24-26-28 ⬇	**ABDOMINALS**	Reg. 14-16-18-20-22-24-26-28 ⬇	Hand to Toes 60
X Sit-Ups 60	Diamond 4-6-8-10-12-14-16 ⬇	Clockwork 60-55-50	Diamond 4-6-8-10-12-14-16 ⬇	X Sit-Ups 60
Crunches 60	Dive Bombers 4-6-8-10-12-14-16 ⬇	Hanging Knee Up 60	Dive Bombers 4-6-8-10-12-14-16 ⬇	Crunches 60
Side Sit-Ups 60	8 Count Body Builders 24	Hanging Side Sit-Up 30	8 Count Body Builders 24	Side Sit-Ups 60
Obliques 60	Take "After" Supplements	Hand to Toe (Short) 60	Take "After" Supplements	Obliques 60
Flutter Kicks 60	Drink 16 oz. of water	Crunches (Short) 60	Drink 16 oz. of water	Flutter Kicks 60
Reverse Crunches 60		Side Sit-Up (Short) 60		Reverse Crunches 60
Knee Bends 60		Obliques (Short) 60		Knee Bends 60
Chest Roll 60		Atomic 50		Chest Roll 60
Take "After" Supplements		Take "After" Supplements		Take "After" Supplements
Drink 16 oz. of water		Drink 16 oz. of water		Drink 16 oz. of water

MEALS / WATER / SUPPLEMENTS

	MONDAY	TUESDAY	WEDNESDAY	THURSDAY	FRIDAY
MEALS	1 2 3 4 / 5	1 2 3 4 / 5	1 2 3 4 / 5	1 2 3 4 / 5	1 2 3 4 / 5
WATER	1 2 3 4 / 5 6 7 8	1 2 3 4 / 5 6 7 8	1 2 3 4 / 5 6 7 8	1 2 3 4 / 5 6 7 8	1 2 3 4 / 5 6 7 8
SUPPLEMENTS Before	3 Electrolyte™ / 1 Energy Plus™	3 Electrolyte™ / 1 Energy Plus™	3 Electrolyte™ / 1 Energy Plus™	3 Electrolyte™ / 1 Energy Plus™	3 Electrolyte™ / 1 Energy Plus™
SUPPLEMENTS After	3 Recover™ / 2 Restore™	3 Recover™ / 2 Restore™	3 Recover™ / 2 Restore™	3 Recover™ / 2 Restore™	3 Recover™ / 2 Restore™

WEEK 12 — ADVANCED LEVEL

✓ MONDAY / /	✓ TUESDAY / /	✓ WEDNESDAY / /	✓ THURSDAY / /	✓ FRIDAY / /
Take "Before" Supplements	Take "Before" Supplements	Take "Before" Supplements	Take "Before" Supplements	Take "Before" Supplements
Drink 16 oz. of water	Drink 16 oz. of water	Drink 16 oz. of water	Drink 16 oz. of water	Drink 16 oz. of water
WARM-UPS	**WARM-UPS**	**WARM-UPS**	**WARM-UPS**	**WARM-UPS**
Jumping Jacks 45	Jumping Jacks 45	Jumping Jacks 45	Jumping Jacks 45	Jumping Jacks 45
Running in Place 60 sec.	Running in Place 60 sec.	Running in Place 60 sec.	Running in Place 60 sec.	Running in Place 60 sec.
Half Jumping Jacks 45	Half Jumping Jacks 45	Half Jumping Jacks 45	Half Jumping Jacks 45	Half Jumping Jacks 45
60–90 sec. Rest	60–90 sec. Rest	60–90 sec. Rest	60–90 sec. Rest	60–90 sec. Rest
STRETCHES	**STRETCHES**	**LEGS**	**STRETCHES**	**STRETCHES**
Bend Overs	Chest	Walking Lunges 40 yds. (5x)	Chest	Bend Overs
Cross Overs	Lat	High Knees 40 yds. (5x)	Lat	Cross Overs
Inner Thigh	Shoulders	Frog Hops 40 yds. (5x)	Shoulders	Inner Thigh
Forward Lunge	Tricep	Star Hops 25	Tricep	Forward Lunge
Side & Oblique	Partner	Mountain Climbers 32	Partner	Side & Oblique
Hurdler	Arm Rotation	**SPRINTS**	Arm Rotation	Hurdler
Butterfly	60–90 sec. Rest	Intervals (Optional)	60–90 sec. Rest	Butterfly
ITB	**UPPER BODY**	12 Laps = 4800 yds.	**UPPER BODY**	ITB
Thigh	Neck Rotations 50		Neck Rotations 50	Thigh
Calf	Back Contractions 50		Back Contractions 50	Calf
60–90 sec. Rest	Swimmer Exercise 50		Swimmer Exercise 50	60–90 sec. Rest
LEGS	Back Lifts 30		Back Lifts 30	**LEGS**
Lunges 50	60–90 sec. Rest		60–90 sec. Rest	Lunges 50
Squats 65	**PULL-UPS**		**PULL-UPS**	Squats 65
Fire Hydrants 45 (Each Side)	Regular 4-6-8-10-12-14-16-18 ⬇		Regular 4-6-8-10-12-14-16-18 ⬇	Fire Hydrants 45 (Each Side)
Mountain Climber 35	Close Grip 2-4-6-8-10-12-14 ⬇		Close Grip 2-4-6-8-10-12-14 ⬇	Mountain Climber 35
The Wall 3:30 min.	Reverse 2-4-6-8-10-12-14 ⬇		Reverse 2-4-6-8-10-12-14 ⬇	The Wall 3:30 min.
60–90 sec. Rest	Commandos 2-4-6-8-10-12 ⬇		Commandos 2-4-6-8-10-12 ⬇	60–90 sec. Rest
CALVES	Behind the Neck 2-4-6-8-10-12 ⬇		Behind the Neck 2-4-6-8-10-12 ⬇	**CALVES**
Straight (Regular) 140	60–90 sec. Rest		60–90 sec. Rest	Straight (Regular) 140
Toe to Toe 140	**BAR DIPS**		**BAR DIPS**	Toe to Toe 140
Heel to Heel 140	Regular 25		Regular 25	Heel to Heel 140
60–90 sec. Rest	60–90 sec. Rest		60–90 sec. Rest	60–90 sec. Rest
ABDOMINALS	**PUSH-UPS**	**ABDOMINALS**	**PUSH-UPS**	**ABDOMINALS**
Hand to Toes 60	Reg. 14-16-18-20-22-24-26-28 ⬇	Clockwork 60-55-50	Reg. 14-16-18-20-22-24-26-28 ⬇	Hand to Toes 60
X Sit-Ups 60	Diamond 4-6-8-10-12-14-16 ⬇	Hanging Knee Up 60	Diamond 4-6-8-10-12-14-16 ⬇	X Sit-Ups 60
Crunches 60	Dive Bombers 4-6-8-10-12-14-16 ⬇	Hanging Side Sit-Up 30	Dive Bombers 4-6-8-10-12-14-16 ⬇	Crunches 60
Side Sit-Ups 60	8 Count Body Builders 24	Hand to Toe (Short) 60	8 Count Body Builders 24	Side Sit-Ups 60
Obliques 60	Take "After" Supplements	Crunches (Short) 60	Take "After" Supplements	Obliques 60
Flutter Kicks 60	Drink 16 oz. of water	Side Sit-Up (Short) 60	Drink 16 oz. of water	Flutter Kicks 60
Reverse Crunches 60		Obliques (Short) 60		Reverse Crunches 60
Knee Bends 60		Atomic 50		Knee Bends 60
Chest Roll 60		Take "After" Supplements		Chest Roll 60
Take "After" Supplements		Drink 16 oz. of water		Take "After" Supplements
Drink 16 oz. of water				Drink 16 oz. of water

MEALS	WATER	MEALS	WATER	MEALS	WATER	MEALS	WATER	MEALS	WATER
1 2 3 4 / 5	1 2 3 4 / 5 6 7 8	1 2 3 4 / 5	1 2 3 4 / 5 6 7 8	1 2 3 4 / 5	1 2 3 4 / 5 6 7 8	1 2 3 4 / 5	1 2 3 4 / 5 6 7 8	1 2 3 4 / 5	1 2 3 4 / 5 6 7 8

SUPPLEMENTS

Before	After	Before	After	Before	After	Before	After	Before	After
3 Electrolyte™ / **1** Energy Plus™	**3** Recover™ / **2** Restore™	**3** Electrolyte™ / **1** Energy Plus™	**3** Recover™ / **2** Restore™	**3** Electrolyte™ / **1** Energy Plus™	**3** Recover™ / **2** Restore™	**3** Electrolyte™ / **1** Energy Plus™	**3** Recover™ / **2** Restore™	**3** Electrolyte™ / **1** Energy Plus™	**3** Recover™ / **2** Restore™

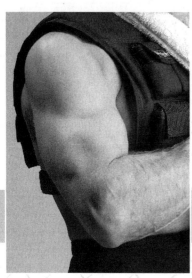

"DON'T STOP! This is only the beginning. Now that you have met your first set of goals, it is time to create new ones."

7

MY AFTER BODY!

1. CONGRATULATIONS!

It wasn't easy, but you did it! You stuck to your guns, even when you didn't always want to, but it has truly paid off. . . .

However, DON'T STOP! This is only the beginning. Now that you have met your first set of goals, it is time to create new ones. *You need to push yourself again to the next level. You can always do better.*

Maybe you have been on the Beginning Level of this program. That's fantastic! But now it is time to go through the program again, at the Intermediate Level or Advanced Level. Once you have finished these milestones, are you done?

Of course not! When you first started this program, you made the decision that you were going to make a paradigm shift or lifestyle change, and you did. So now is not the time to quit. Even if you are already at the Advanced Level, you still need to maintain your current body. *You have worked too hard to go backward!*

By now you will have already started to see other aspects of your life begin to change. You look better, feel younger, and have more confidence. *Make the commitment today to never stop. Keep pushing yourself to the next level.* Also, push those whom you care about as well. After all, if they don't feel and look like you do, they will not want to go with you on your next cruise!

2. WHERE ARE YOU NOW?

As a closing to this session, retake the fitness test again to see how much you have improved. As you do this, *use your new numbers as the benchmark for your next level of progression.* We wish you good luck as you take it to the next level!

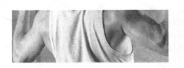

FITNESS REEVALUATION

EXERCISES (Regular)	Total Max Reps	Beginning Level	Intermediate Level	Advanced Level
Old Push-Ups				
New Push-Ups				
Difference				
Old Crunches				
New Crunches				
Difference				
Old Lunges				
New Lunges				
Difference				
Old Bar Dips				
New Bar Dips				
Difference				
Flutter Kicks				
Flutter Kicks				
Difference				
Calf Raises				
Calf Raises				
Difference				

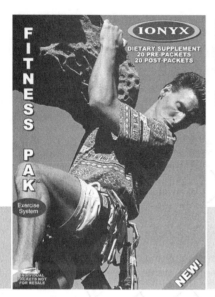

20 Pre-Packets and 20 Post-Packets in a Fitness Pak have been created to fully support this workout.

IONYX CUTTING-EDGE MINERAL SUPPLEMENTATION

Proper supplementation of key nutrients is critical for one's body to function at peak performance while exercising. When you perspire, you lose more than water to cool your overheated body. You also lose important electrolytes (essential minerals) that help control fluid levels in the body, maintain normal pH levels, and ensure the correct electric potential between nerve cells, which enables the proper transmission of nerve signals.

Minerals are a key to a person's overall good health because 95 percent of the body's daily functions require them. Our bodies cannot produce minerals, so they must be ingested through the foods and liquids we consume. Unfortunately, eating the right foods is no longer good enough because the mineral content of our foods is on the decline. If you compare the 1963 and 1997 United States Department of Agriculture Nutrition Tables, most of the trace and essential minerals in our fruits, vegetables, and meats have decreased considerably. The loss varies from 20 to 85 percent on any given mineral, and wisdom tells you that supplementation is necessary to avoid deficiency, especially if you work out.

I never realized how important minerals were until I started using a phenomenal electrolyte product from IONYX International, Inc., which uses a unique formula that replaces the electrolytes lost during intense workouts. I take their electrolyte supplement every day before I exercise, and I've had amazing results. I found that I have more energy during the workout and am able to perform longer without the muscle fatigue that normally kicks in. That enables me to press the fatigue threshold and perform at a higher level. I also discovered that my muscle recovery was much quicker, since I was replenishing the minerals my body sweats out.

When I compared the IONYX products to others on the market, they have no equal. The minerals from IONYX are the most bio-available because they are the smallest in size. They have natural assimilative properties, so they do not need to be put into a solution or have other ingredients attached to them to be absorbed into your body. They have pH balancing characteristics that are more concentrated than other supplements.

I am not the only one who has seen amazing results using the IONYX supplements. George

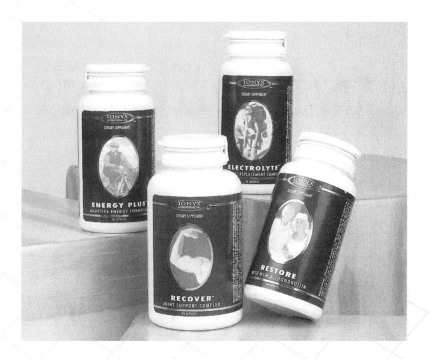

Curtis, the head athletic trainer for the athletic programs at Brigham Young University, put his athletes on the IONYX supplements. After they became the only university that had all five fall sports programs ranked in the national top 20, here's what Curtis had to say:

"We have had an ongoing problem for years trying to find the right combination of electrolytes to take with our combination of drinks. It has been a real difficult task. We have tried all kinds of combinations, but this spring when we tried IONYX products it was great to see how much they eased the problem with some of the chronic problems athletes had. We will be exclusively buying the IONYX Electrolyte supplements over other previous products."

Another individual who has had great results using IONYX supplements with his athletes is David Houle, head coach for Mountain View High School and national high school Coach of the Year 2000 and 2002, who has won 57 state championships throughout his career coaching basketball and track and field. When he gave the IONYX products to his kids, listen to these results:

"For the past couple of months I have been sampling a product by the name of IONYX. I have had athletes from various sports that I coach try this product, and they have found it to be very beneficial. It is a natural product that helps kids with their stamina. I have witnessed some of my athletes break personal, state, and national records using IONYX products. Clearly, I am excited about this product line and what it can do to help the quality of our everyday lives."

If you do not replenish your electrolytes while exercising, your body may suffer fatigue, low stamina, muscle cramping, lack of recovery, and even invite disaster! The electrolyte supplement from IONYX is ideal for anyone who experiences high fluid and electrolyte loss, and I recommend it completely.

> For more information about these electrolyte supplements or to find out how to purchase IONYX products, please refer to my Web site at www.masterlevelfitness.com.

PRE-WORKOUT SUPPLEMENTS

ELECTROLYTE™ Mineral Replacement Complex: When individuals perspire, they lose more than water to cool their overheated body. They also lose precious electrolytes (essential minerals). Our unique formula replaces not only the common electrolytes needed for peak performance, but the ionic minerals that are commonly overlooked when electrolyte replacement is considered. If individuals do not replenish their electrolytes, their body may suffer fatigue, low stamina, muscle cramping, lack of recovery, and even invite disaster! This complex is ideal for those individuals who need to enhance their sports performance, or when they experience high fluid and electrolyte loss. (Take 3 capsules before each workout.)

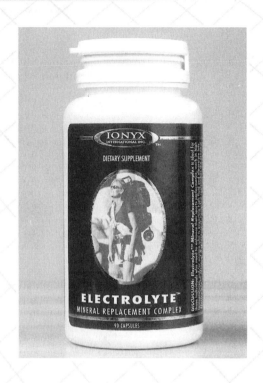

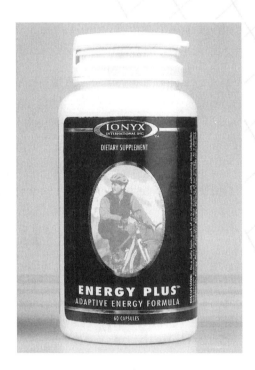

ENERGY PLUS™ Adaptive Energy Formula: This complex increases one's energy level during stressful and intense workouts. Siberian and Korean Ginseng help one's body to withstand adverse physical and mental conditions during cases of weakness, exhaustion, and tiredness, while improving mental alertness. Guarana provides extra stamina and endurance, increases strength, reduces fatigue, and helps dispose the body of lactic acid, which builds up in the muscles and causes muscle fatigue. Vitamin B complex is essential for maintaining energy levels and ensuring long-lasting performance. (Take 1 capsule before each workout.)

POST-WORKOUT SUPPLEMENTS

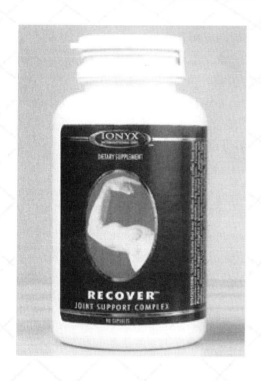

RECOVER™ Joint Support Complex: When one is constantly building and developing stamina and endurance, it is critical to not overlook the importance of fortifying one's body with the nutrients needed for optimum joint wellness. Common "wear and tear" can be minimized with proper supplementation. Glucosamine, in combination with other supportive ingredients in this formula, nourish one's body so it can repair itself and return its joints to proper health. While many drugs are used to fight against joint discomfort, they regrettably only target the symptoms and do very little to address the actual problem. Glucosamine, on the other hand, is a natural aminomonosaccaride found in high concentrated amounts in healthy joints, connective tissues, and cartilage. As a result, this formula is the better long-term choice for healthy joints. (Take 3 capsules after each workout.)

RESTORE™ With MSM & Chondroitin: This unique formula is a synergistic blend of MSM, Chondroitin, and other beneficial herbs, which provide the building blocks for the body to repair its joints. MSM assists the body in healing and repairing many of its tissues, especially those at risk of repeated damage. Chondroitin is a major constituent found in cartilage that helps form holes within the matrix of one's joints, which the body fills with water, creating a spongy shock absorber for the joints. (Take 2 capsules after each workout.)

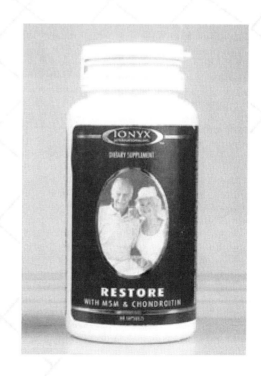

IONYX ICE™

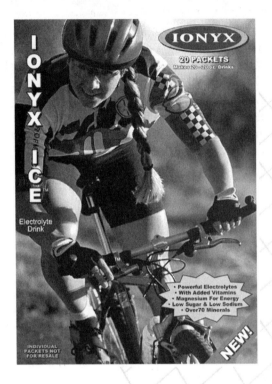

IONYX has created what I believe is the most cutting-edge electrolyte drink on the market today. Besides providing the hydration so critical for cooling down your body during a workout, IONYX ICE™ Electrolyte Drink replenishes the essential electrolytes and minerals lost through perspiring and helps maintain your stamina, endurance, and overall performance. And it is the only electrolyte drink that I am aware of that also has 100 percent of the daily recommended dose of Vitamin C, an array of B-vitamins for energy, and the magnesium that helps curtail cramping and plays a critical role in ATP (energy) production in your body. IONYX ICE™ Electrolyte Drink tastes fantastic, yet contains half as much sodium and sugar as many other popular sports drinks! If you are looking for a sports drink to enhance your performance, replace your electrolytes and trace minerals, and fortify your vitamin intake, I recommend IONYX ICE™ Electrolyte Drink. (Each box makes 20 twenty-ounce drinks. Take before, during, and after your workout.)

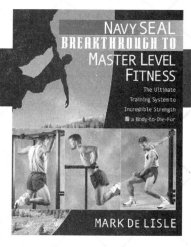
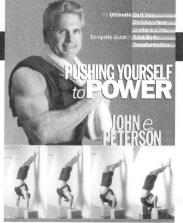

NOTES

NOTES

NOTES

NOTES

NOTES